Flight Medical Provider:
A Ground and Flight Critical Care Guide

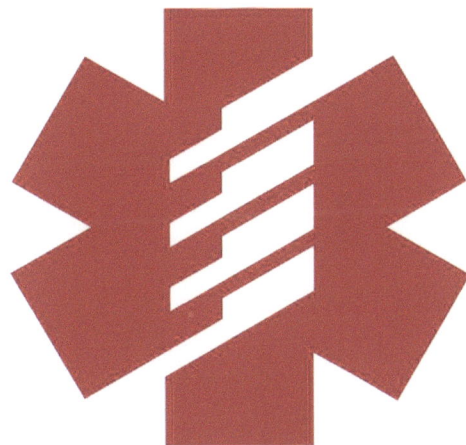

IMPACT
EMS TRAINING

Gwenny Lawson, BA, BSN, CFRN, CTRN, RN
Michael Carunchio, MS, FP-C, TP-C

KN⦿WFULLY
LEARNING GROUP

Contributors:

Jaren Jarrell, NRP, FP-C
Richard D. Maricle, BAAS, NRP, FP-C
George A. Taylor, NRP, FP-C

Reviewers:

Jaren Jarrell, NRP, FP-C
Richard D. Maricle, BAAS, NRP, FP-C
Allyson Moschera, NRP
Sarah C. Motley, BSN, RN, NREMT-B
George A. Taylor, NRP, FP-C

Medical Director:

Salim Rezaie, MD, FACEP
Emergency Medicine & Internal Medicine
Greater San Antonio Emergency Physicians (GSEP)
Founder/Creator/Editor/Author of R.E.B.E.L. EM and REBEL REVIEWS

Cover Design:

Allyson Moschera, NRP

Table of Contents

Dear Reader,

Thank you for entrusting the **Impact EMS Training** team with your continuing prehospital and critical care education. Learning new and complex information, turning it into knowledge, and applying it to patient care and prehospital operations can be intimidating. It is our mission to help guide you through the learning process.

Impact EMS Training takes your pursuit of knowledge very seriously and we are both confident and proud of the information that you will find in these pages. This book is a product of hundreds of hours of research, content writing, meticulous reference checking, peer editing, and revisions. It has been independently audited by expert educators and industry accreditation consultants and has been reviewed by physicians and other specialty experts.

We believe the content in this book is maximized when used as an adjunct to our Flight Medical Provider™ (FMP) course. The sequence of the book directly mirrors the course and we have allotted ample space for notes in the margins. Later, go back and study both the information in the text and the notes you took in the book during the FMP course. I think you'll find it to be a rich resource for years to come!

Remember: this book is just the foundation for your learning endeavor. Take our FMP course. Use different types of resources like podcasts, videos, and online emergency and critical care websites like RebelEM to continuously supplement your knowledge and become a well-rounded critical care paramedic or nurse.

We pride ourselves in being dependable industry members who continue to work in the field doing the job every day as prehospital and critical care nurses and paramedics just like so many of you. Please reach out to us with questions; we routinely personally respond to emails and enjoy maintaining that relationship with you, our students.

Our kick-ass team of instructors love meeting our students at in-person courses and in our livestream sessions. Please visit our website at www.ImpactEMS.com to reserve your seat at one of our events!

To the brilliant minds that collaborated on this book, thank you for your hard work and hours spent buried in books, glued to a computer screen, and interviewing experts. I am wildly proud of every single one of you and admire your passionate pursuit of excellence!

Be safe and stay well,

Gwenny Lawson
Director of Education
Impact EMS Training

IMPACT EMS TRAINING

History

EMT & Fire Training was created in 2009 to provide comprehensive Emergency Medical Technician (EMT) training to individuals who struggled to fit traditional Emergency Medical Services (EMS) programs into their demanding schedules. In 2011, IA MED was founded with a distinct mission: to revolutionize EMS education and transform how students are instructed, focusing on flight and critical care medicine.

Over the years, both companies have significantly contributed to the industry, leaving a lasting impact. Recognizing the synergy and advantage that merging these organizations would bring, Knowfully Learning Group acquired both EMT & Fire Training and IA MED.

The combined strength of EMT & Fire Training, IA MED, and Knowfully Learning Group represents a powerful force committed to driving innovation and shaping the future of EMS education. As a result, we are uniquely positioned to serve the diverse needs of the industry and empower individuals with the skills and knowledge required to excel in their roles.

With a shared vision and a relentless pursuit of excellence, our united organization is poised to profoundly impact prehospital care and advance the quality of care provided to patients worldwide.

At **Impact EMS Training**, we pride ourselves on offering a holistic and all-encompassing suite of services catering to our students' needs at every stage of their educational journey. Our programs encompass various meticulously designed courses that will lay a solid foundation for a promising EMS career. With our ever-growing catalog of continuing education programs, we can provide lifelong learning and professional growth opportunities.

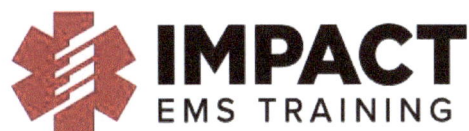

Chapter 1: Advanced Airway Management

"In my opinion and experience, most 'difficult' airways in emergency medicine/critical care are 'inadequately prepared for' airways."
-Cliff Reid, Prehospital Critical Care Physician & Educator

Importance of Airway Management
- Life ending or altering injuries to patients
- Mental burden on staff
- Costly legal settlements
- "Do It For Drew" campaign

AIRWAY anatomy

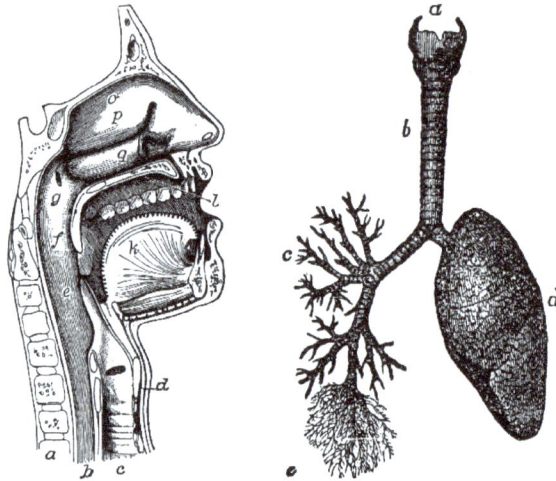

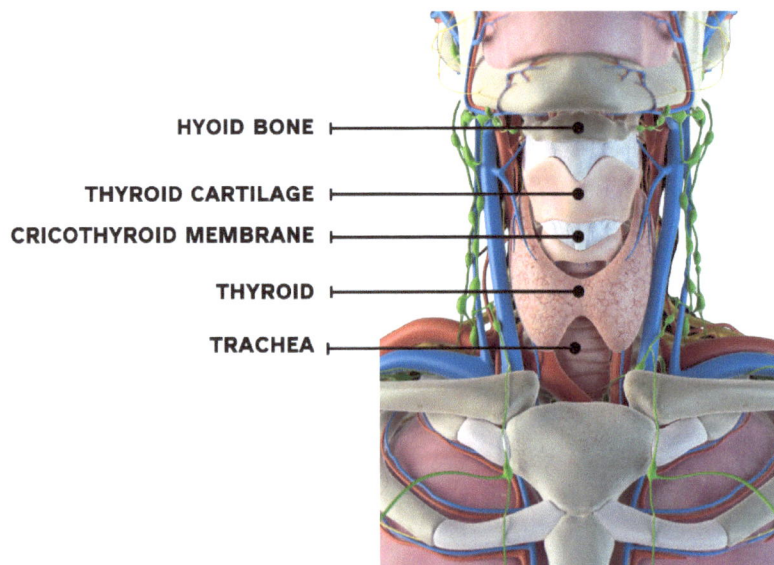

HYOID BONE

THYROID CARTILAGE

CRICOTHYROID MEMBRANE

THYROID

TRACHEA

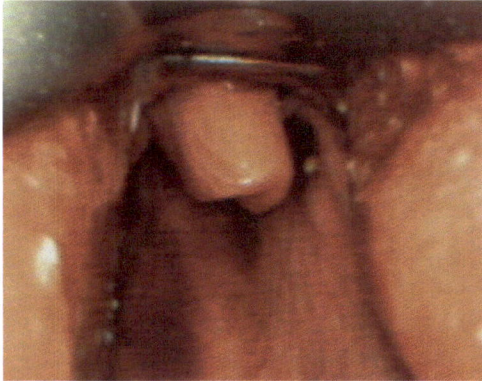

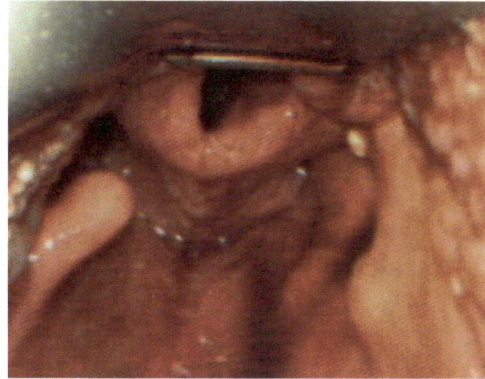

Photos from a CMAC blade during intubation by Chris Smetana

AIRWAY ASSESSMENT

- **Primary assessment or MARCHE**
- **Patency of airway**
    - **Speech**
    - **Mentation**
    - **General appearance**
    - **Respiratory pattern & effort**
    - **Lung sounds**
    - **Airway contaminants**
    - **Immediate or potential life threats**
- **Respiratory Patterns**
    - **Rate**
    - **Depth**
    - **Regularity**
    - **Effectiveness**
    - **Indicative of pathology**
        - **Kussmaul's**
        - **Biot's**
        - **Cheyne-Stokes**
        - **Apneustic**

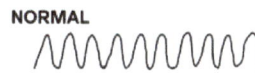

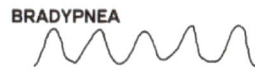

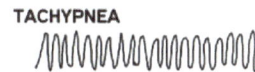

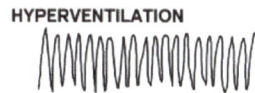

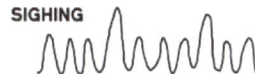

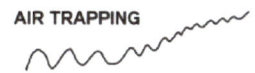

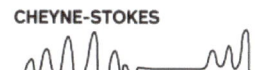

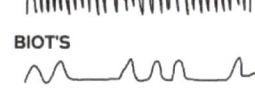

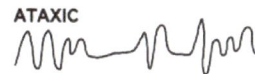

Pediatric Airway Assessment

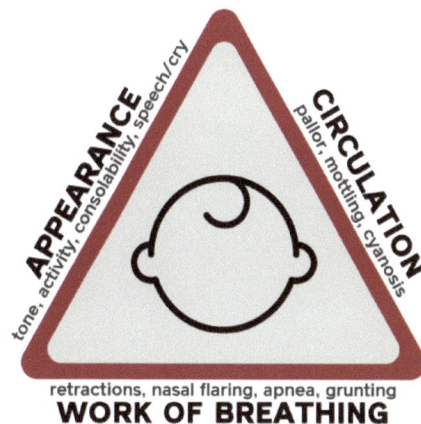

9

Airway Interventions[2]

- **Supplementary oxygen**
  - Nasal cannula
  - Non-rebreather mask
  - Bag valve mask: use PEEP valve and capnography
    - Two thumbs up technique

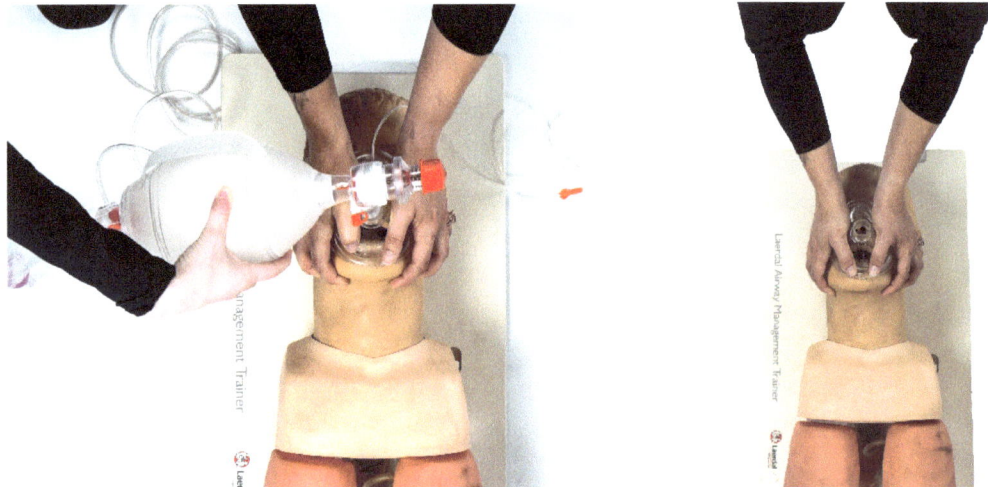

  - **Extraglottic airways**[2]
    - Supraglottic: creates mask seal around laryngeal opening

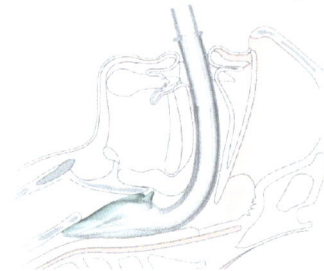

    - Retroglottic: seated posterior to glottis in proximal esophagus

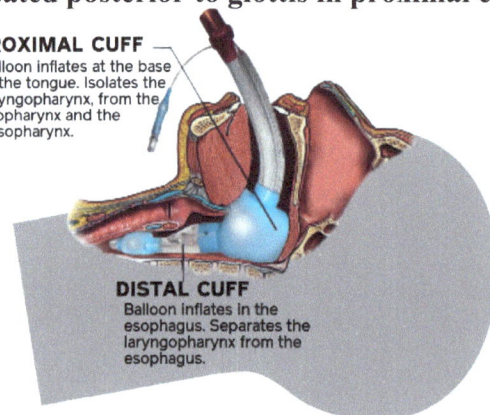

PROXIMAL CUFF
Balloon inflates at the base of the tongue. Isolates the laryngopharynx, from the oropharynx and the nasopharynx.

DISTAL CUFF
Balloon inflates in the esophagus. Separates the laryngopharynx from the esophagus.

- High flow nasal cannula[4]
  - **Heated**
  - **Humidified**
  - **Replaces dead space with oxygen**
  - **Up to 60LPM**

Indication for Intubation
- **Failure to oxygenate or ventilate with less invasive interventions**
- **Predicted clinical course**
- **Failure to protect airway**
- **Patient or crew safety**

PREPARATION

Monitor w/capno, IVs, resuscitation/pressors
Supplies: ETT w/syringe, bougie, SGA, cric kit, suction,
VL/DL on, tube tamer, OG/NG, RSI meds

PRE-OXYGENATE

8 vital capacity breaths w/O via NC & NRB
BVM w/PEEP and passive O via NC @15 LPM

POSITION

Ramp to 30°, ear to sternal notch, pad shoulders
of pediatrics

PRE-TREATMENT & PARALYSIS

Sedation & analgesia FIRST, then paralytic
Confirm all doses & volumes with partner

PLACEMENT W/PROOF

Lead with suction, verbalize visualization of cords,
place ETT, inflate the cuff, ventilate patient,
waveform ETCO2, bilateral lung sounds, CXR

POST-INTUBATION MANAGEMENT

Secure ETT, place OG/NG, apply mechanical
ventilator, ongoing sedation & analgesia, ensure
adequate blood pressure

AIRWAY CHECKLIST

- ☐ MONITOR & IVS
- ☐ RESUSCITATE
  fluid, blood, pressors
- ☐ PRE-OXYGENATE
  NRB+NC or BVM w/PEEP & 2 thumbs up
- ☐ POSITION
  ramp, ear to sternal notch
- ☐ DIFFICULT AIRWAY INDICATORS
  - Hypoxemia
  - Extreme of size
  - Anatomic disruption
  - Vomit or airway contaminant
  - Exsanguination
  - Neck injury
- ☐ EQUIPMENT READY
  - Bougie
  - Suction
  - Laryngoscope
  - ETT tube w/syringe attached
  - OG tube
  - Tube holder under patient's neck
  - Back up airway
  - Cric kit
  - Medication drawn up & confirmed w/partner

- ☐ INDUCTION AGENT ADMINISTERED
- ☐ PARALYTIC AGENT ADMINISTERED
- ☐ INTUBATE
  - Lead w/suction
- ☐ CONFIRM ETT PLACEMENT
  - Visualization of cords
  - Waveform capnography
  - Bilateral breath sounds & absence of epigastric sounds
- ☐ SECURE TUBE
- ☐ INSERT GASTRIC DECOMPRESSION TUBE
- ☐ CONFIRM ETT PLACEMENT
  - Mechanical ventilation
- ☐ SEDATION & ANALGESIA

HEAVEN Criteria[3]

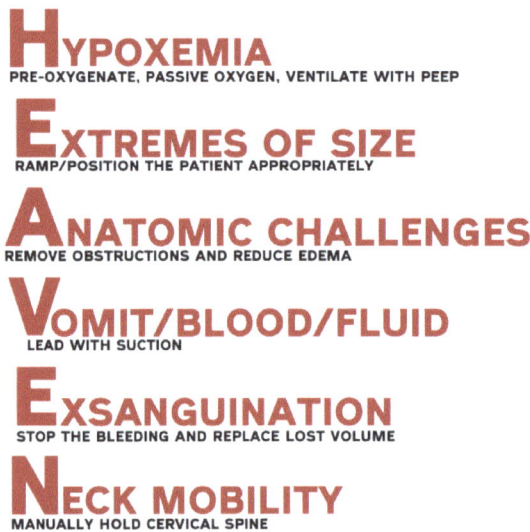

HYPOXEMIA
PRE-OXYGENATE, PASSIVE OXYGEN, VENTILATE WITH PEEP

EXTREMES OF SIZE
RAMP/POSITION THE PATIENT APPROPRIATELY

ANATOMIC CHALLENGES
REMOVE OBSTRUCTIONS AND REDUCE EDEMA

VOMIT/BLOOD/FLUID
LEAD WITH SUCTION

EXSANGUINATION
STOP THE BLEEDING AND REPLACE LOST VOLUME

NECK MOBILITY
MANUALLY HOLD CERVICAL SPINE

Rapid Sequence Intubation: back-to-back administration of sedative and paralytic to facilitate emergency endotracheal intubation

Delayed Sequence Intubation: time between sedative and paralytic to oxygenate and achieve hemodynamic optimization[1]

Delayed Sequence Intubation

Preoxygenation and passive oxygenation lengthens the safe apnea period
- **Spontaneous breathing patient:**
  - **8 vital capacity breaths on 15L NRB**
- **Apneic patient:**
  - **BVM with PEEP using 2-thumbs up**

Passive oxygenation: >15L via regular nasal cannula

Resuscitate[1,2]
- **Achieve hemodynamic stability**
  - **MAP > 65mmHg**
  - **CVP 8–12mmHg**
  - **Improve mental status**
- **Correct hypotension**
  - **Blood loss = blood products**
  - **Fluid loss = isotonic fluids**
  - **Loss of vascular tone = pressors**

Positioning/Ramping: ear to sternal notch with HOB 30°

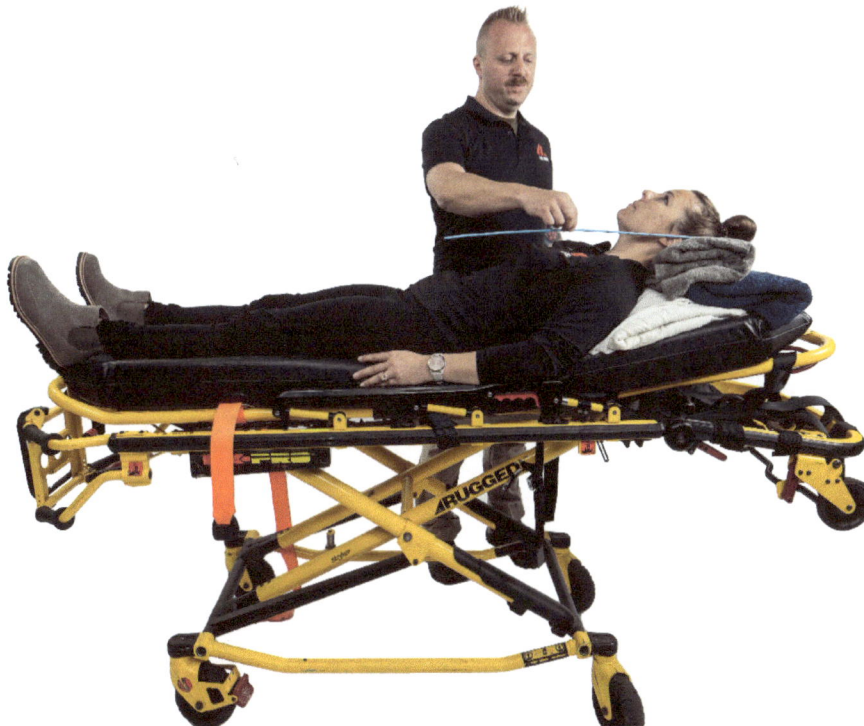

Intubation Equipment Preparation

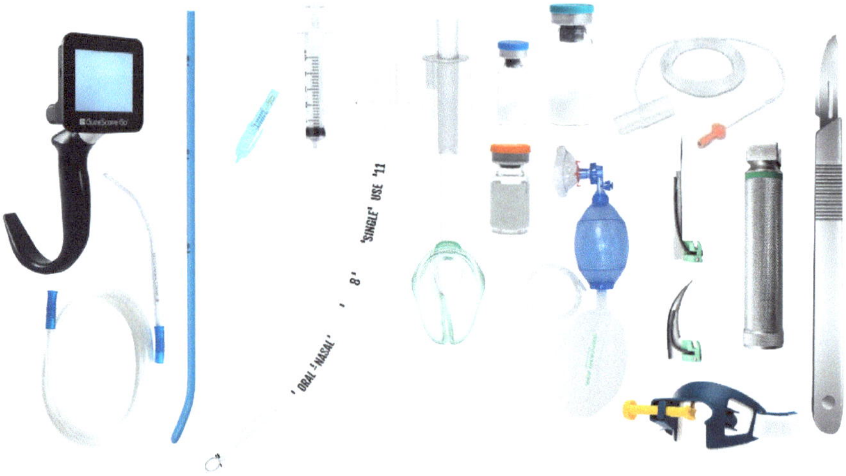

Apneic Oxygenation
- Goal: to extend the safe apnea period that occurs during endotracheal intubation
- REGULAR nasal cannula 15-25LPM
- For ease of removal post intubation, loop oxygen tubing under patient's ears and cinch at the top of the head

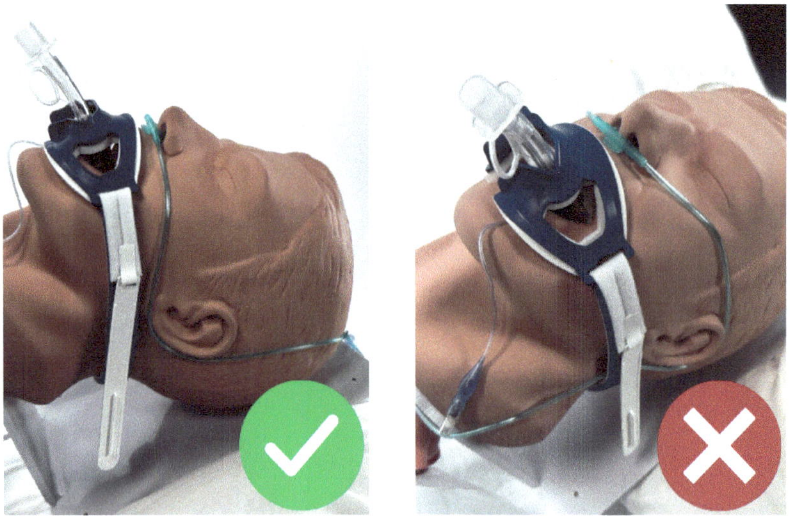

Direct Laryngoscopy (DL)
- Inexpensive
- Easy to maintain
- Not affected prohibitively by airway contaminants

Video Laryngoscopy (VL)
- Facilitates visualization of oropharyngeal structures
- Camera can be rendered useless by airway contaminants

Endotracheal Tubes

- **Size 2.5mm-9.0mm: lumen diameter**
  - **Flow is affected exponentially by tube diameter, thus larger tubes facilitate improved air flow**
  - **Leave ETT in the package as long as possible to reduce introduction of microbes into trachea**
- **Pre-attach syringe filled with air or manometer**

Pediatric Endotracheal Tubes[1]
- **ETT size: [(age in years ÷ 4) + 4]**
- **Use cuffed ETTs for all but "youngest infants"**

Endotracheal Tube Introducers[1]
- **Curved tip is designed to guide the user into anterior airway**
- **Improves first pass success rate without significantly increasing time or incidence of hypoxia**
- **Bougie tube exchange**
- **Technique variation: Kiwi technique**
  - **More practical for single provider**
  - **Contaminates ETT**
  - **Diminishes articulation ability of bougie**

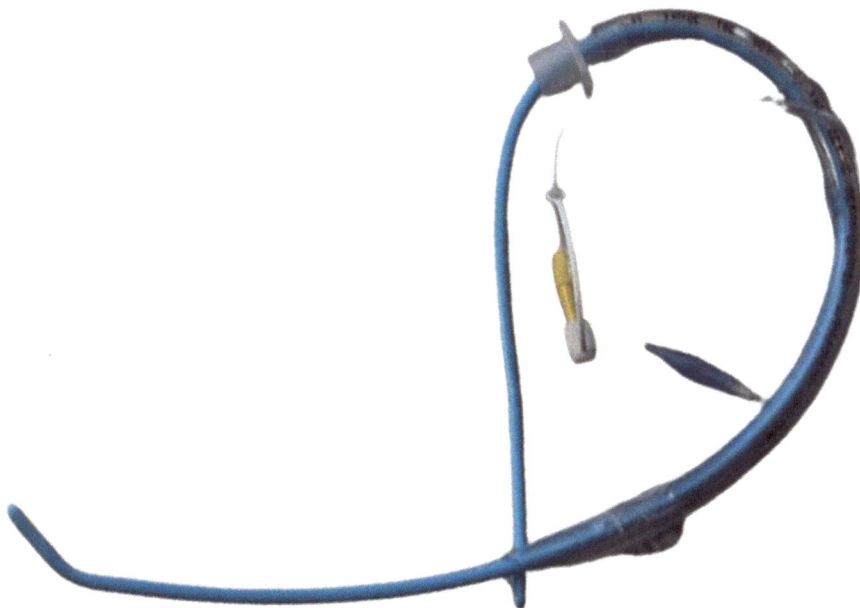

SALAD Technique

- **Lead with suction to clear oropharynx prior to blade insertion**
- **Park suction in esophagus on left side of mouth**
- **Insert blade with suction still in place**
- **Goals**
    - **Prevent video laryngoscope contamination**
    - **Prevent introducing airway contaminants into lungs during endotracheal tube insertion**

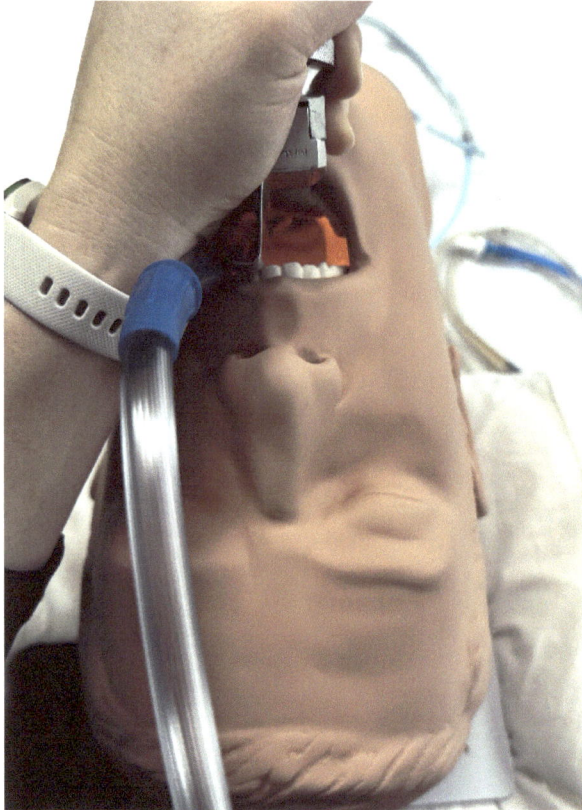

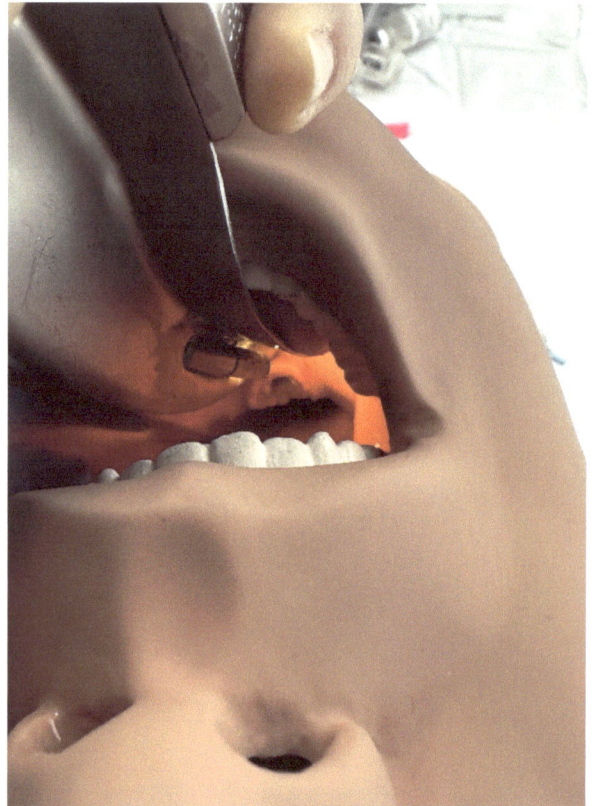

ETT Cuff Pressure[5]
- Safe adult pressure 20-30 cm H_2O
- <20 cm H_2O increases risk of ventilator-associated pneumonia by 400%
- 30-50 cm H_2O is associated with impaired tracheal capillary perfusion

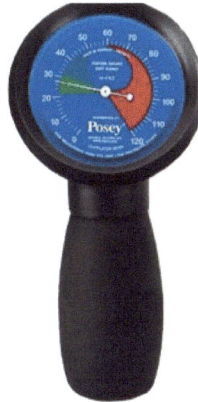

Placement Confirmation: Endotracheal
- Direct visualization: proximal end of cuff 1-2cm beyond cords[7]
- Auscultation: absence of epigastric, presence of bilateral
- Placement in trachea: $ETCO_2$
  - Quantitative
  - Qualitative

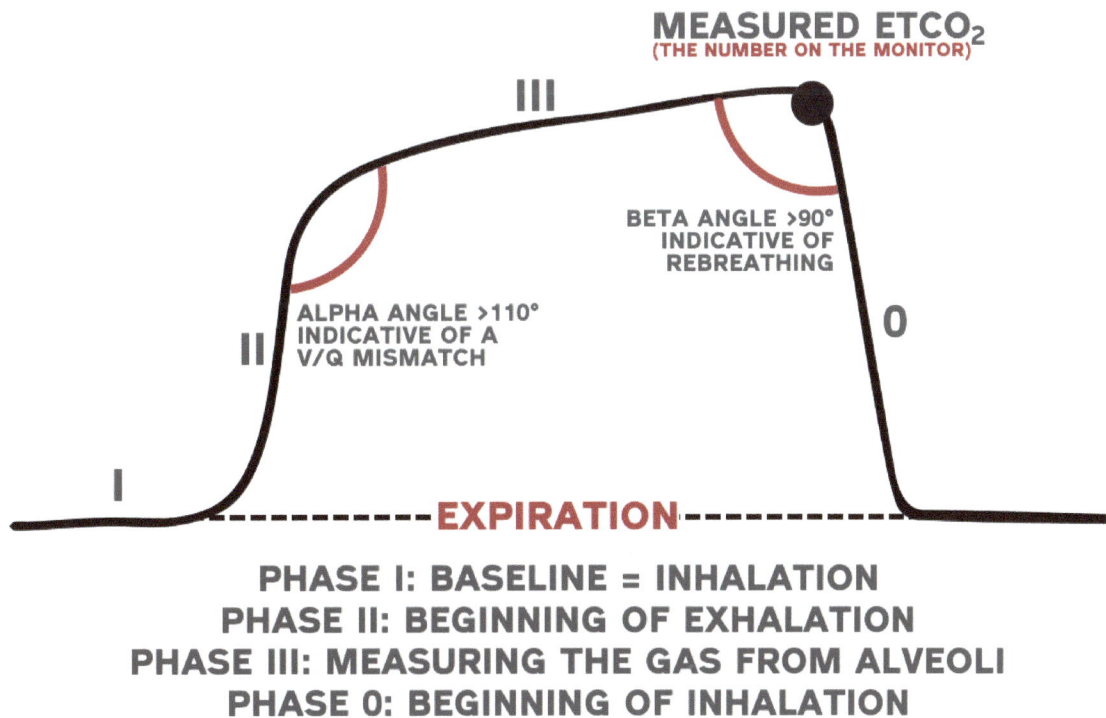

MEASURED $ETCO_2$
(THE NUMBER ON THE MONITOR)

III

BETA ANGLE >90°
INDICATIVE OF
REBREATHING

ALPHA ANGLE >110°
INDICATIVE OF A
V/Q MISMATCH

II

0

I

EXPIRATION

PHASE I: BASELINE = INHALATION
PHASE II: BEGINNING OF EXHALATION
PHASE III: MEASURING THE GAS FROM ALVEOLI
PHASE 0: BEGINNING OF INHALATION

Placement Confirmation: Depth
- **Chest x-ray**
    - **5cm above carina (+/-2cm)**
    - **T2-T4**
    - **Collar bones junction**

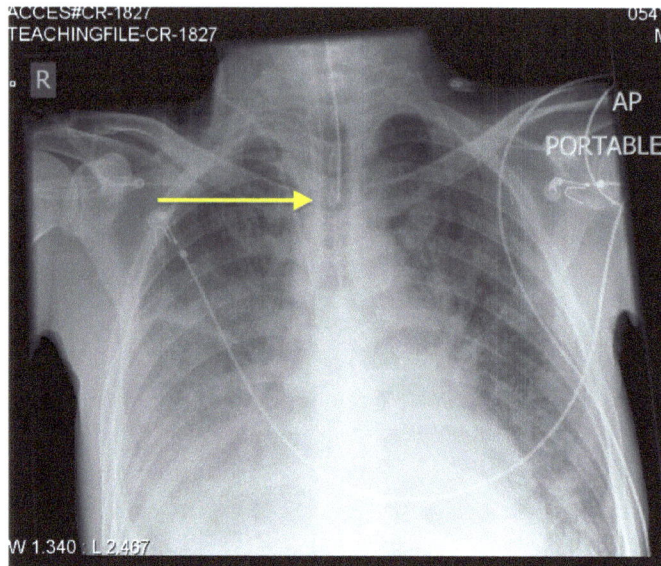

DSI Pharmacology
- **Pre-treatment**
- **Analgesics**
- **Induction (sedation)**
- **Paralytics**
- **Post-intubation management**

ALL MEDICATIONS (dose and volume) SHOULD BE CONFIRMED WITH BOTH PARTNERS BEFORE ADMINISTRATION

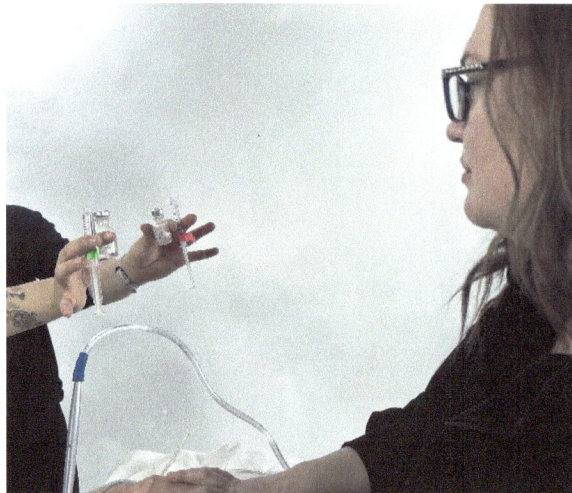

Atropine (anticholinergic)

- **Dose:** 0.02mg/kg/dose IV, may repeat once
- **Minimum dose:** 0.1mg
- **Max:** 0.5mg/dose
- **Inhibits action of acetylcholinesterase on autonomic effectors innervated by postganglionic nerves, thus preventing vagal stimulation induced bradycardia during intubation**

Etomidate (sedative, amnestic)
- **Dose:** 0.3mg/kg
- **Onset:** 30 seconds
- **Duration:** 5-10 minutes
- **Anxiolytic sedative and hypnotic agent well suited induction agent for RSI due to its minimal cardiovascular side effects**

Fentanyl (synthetic opioid analgesic)
- **Dose:** 1-3mcg/kg
- **Drip:** 1-2mcg/kg/hr
- **Duration of action:** 30-60 minutes
- **Opiate receptor agonist inhibits pain pathways; causes peripheral vasodilation by depressing the responsiveness of the alpha-adrenergic receptors; decreases preload, afterload, and may also decrease myocardial oxygen demand**

Ketamine (dissociative anesthetic, analgesic)
- **Induction dose:** 1-2mg/kg
- **Pain dose:** 0.1-0.25mg/kg
- **Drip:** 5-20mcg/kg/min
- **Duration of action (IV):** 5-15 minutes
- **Produces dissociative anesthesia, blocks NMDA receptor, provides sedation and analgesia**
- **Also provides bronchodilatory effects**

Midazolam (benzodiazepine)
- **Induction dose:** 0.1mg/kg
- **Drip:** 20-100mcg/kg/hr
- **Duration of action:** 60-90 minutes
- **Acts at the level of the limbic, thalamic, and hypothalamic regions of the CNS by enhancing effects of neurotransmitter GABA; Decreases nerve cell activity in all regions of CNS, causes retrograde amnesia**

Propofol (general anesthetic)
- Initial dose: 40mg every 10sec to desired effect
- Drip: 5-200mcg/kg/min
- Duration of action: 3-5 minutes
- Short acting hypnotic that produces amnesia <u>but has NO analgesic properties</u>
- Can cause profound hypotension

Succinylcholine (Depolarizing neuromuscular blockade)
- Dose: 1.5mg/kg
- Onset: 30-45 seconds
- Duration: 5-10 minutes
- Ultra-short acting, depolarizing skeletal muscle relaxant
- Has many contraindications!
- Malignant hyperthermia

Rocuronium (nondepolarizing neuromuscular blocker)
- Dose: 0.6-1.2mg/kg
- Onset: 45-120 seconds
- Duration: 30-90 minutes
- Prevents neuromuscular transmission by blocking the effect of acetylcholine at the myoneural junction

Vecuronium (nondepolarizing neuromuscular blocker)
- Dose: 0.1mg/kg MAX: 10mg
- Onset: 30-60 seconds
- Duration: 25-40 minutes
- Prevents neuromuscular transmission by competing for cholinergic receptors at the motor endplate

Pharmacokinetics in Hemodynamically Unstable Patients

induction **HALF DOSE** + paralytic **DOUBLE DOSE** + **PRESSORS**

Post intubation management[2]
- Gastric decompression
- Sedation & pain management
  - RASS -5 (unarousable) to +4 (combative)
- Tube securement
- Mechanical ventilation

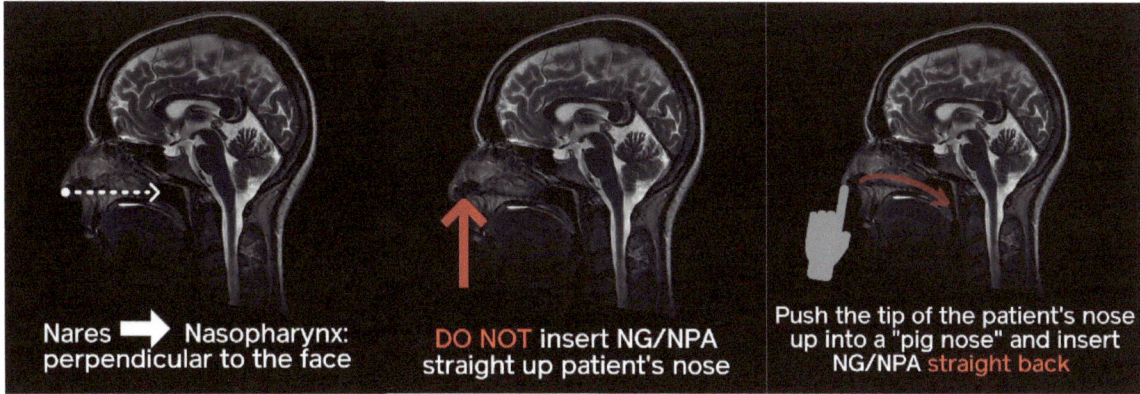

Nares ➡ Nasopharynx: perpendicular to the face

DO NOT insert NG/NPA straight up patient's nose

Push the tip of the patient's nose up into a "pig nose" and insert NG/NPA straight back

Airway Algorithms

Difficult Airway[2]

- **Tools guide the crew to predict complications to endotracheal intubation, mitigate risks, and effectively plan**
  - **Anatomic**
  - **Physiologic**

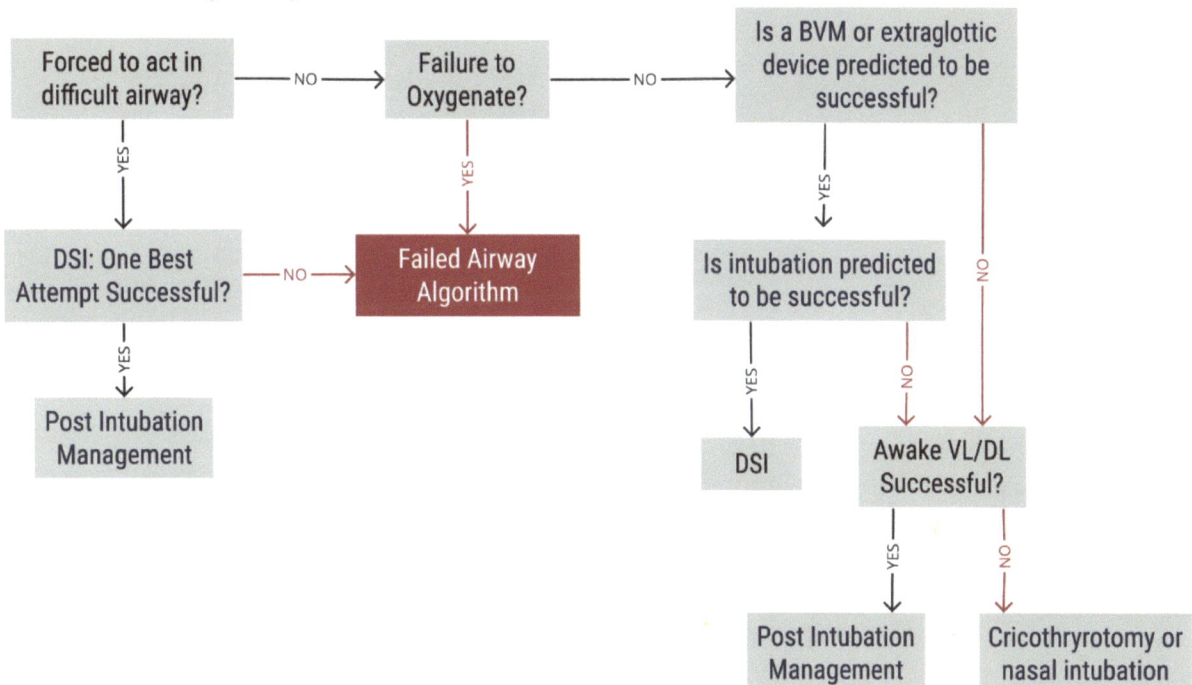

Failed Airway[2]
Failure to oxygenate, failure to ventilate
- **Failure to maintain oxygenation during or after 1+ endotracheal intubation attempts**
- **Three failed attempts at endotracheal intubation by the most qualified intubator**
- **Forced to act situation**

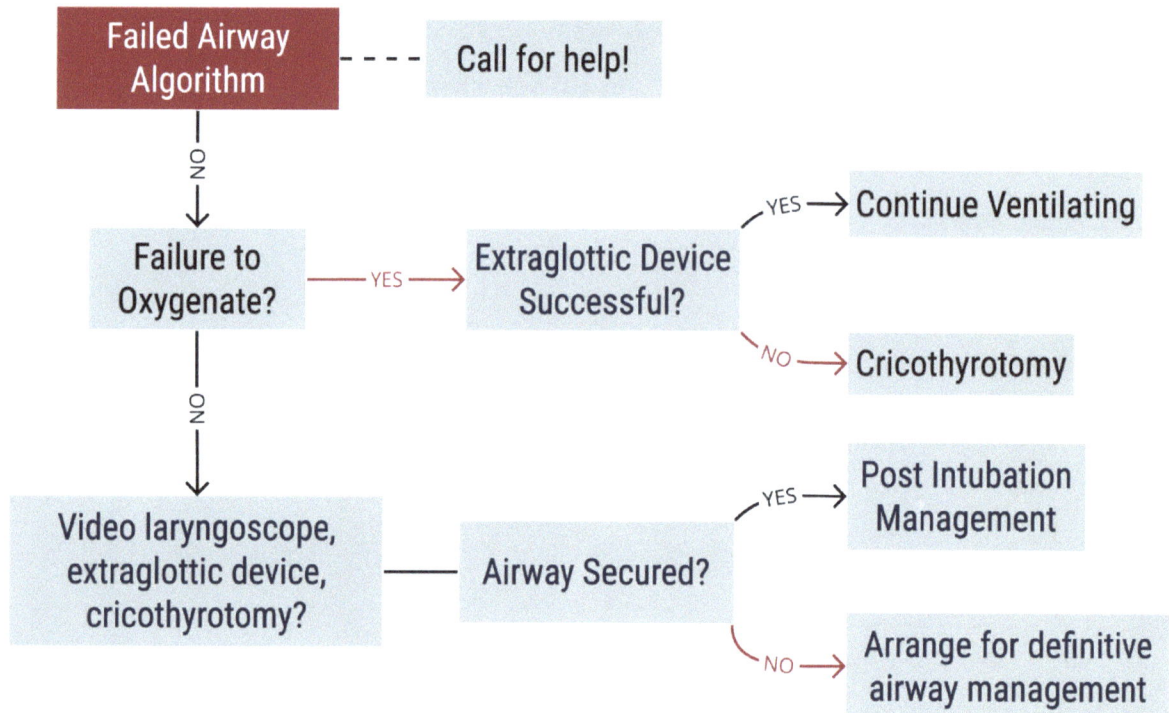

Considerations for Managing the Airway in Special Populations

Bariatric Patients[2]
- **Very high risk for rapid desaturation during intubation**
- **Increased work to distribute oxygen to tissues**
- **Large abdominal contents can impede diaphragm**
    - **DO NOT lay these patients flat**
        - **Hypoxia**
        - **Hypotension**

Obstetric Patients[2]
- **Increased minute ventilation, rate**
    - **Mild respiratory alkalosis: ETCO$_2$ 30mmHg**
    - **MUST maintain SpO$_2$ >95%**
- **Chronic respiratory diseases worsen in pregnancy**

Pediatric Patients[2]

Leading cause of pediatric cardiac arrest is HYPOXIA

- Remove the child's clothing to assess work of breathing
- Infants are obligate nose breathers
- Heads are larger in proportion to bodies than adults
    - Pad the shoulders (NOT the head) to achieve neutral neck position

Patients with Anatomic Abnormalities

- Down syndrome, Turner syndrome: expect anomalous airway
- Cervical fixation: hold manual spinal immobilization, open c-collar
- Edema: go down a half to full size ETT

Surgical Cricothyrotomy

- Most difficult part: the decision to do it
- Contraindications: NONE
    - But red flags to be aware of
        - Anticoagulated patients
        - Goiters or tumors

Needle Cricothyrotomy Equipment

- 14g catheter-over-needle system
- 3mL syringe, plunger removed
- 7.0 ETT adapter
- BVM with ETCO$_2$

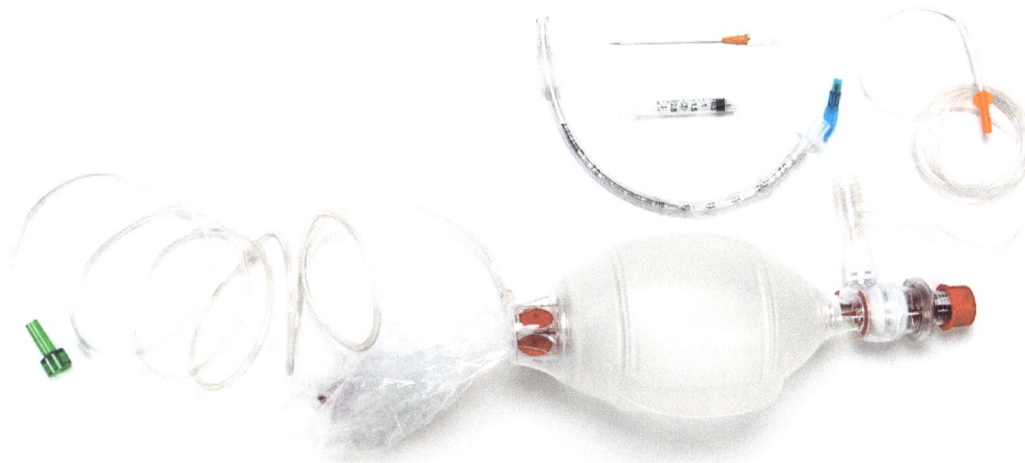

Needle Cricothyrotomy Ventilation Set-Up Order:
BVM > ETCO$_2$ > 7.0 ETT adapter > 3mL syringe > 14g angiocath

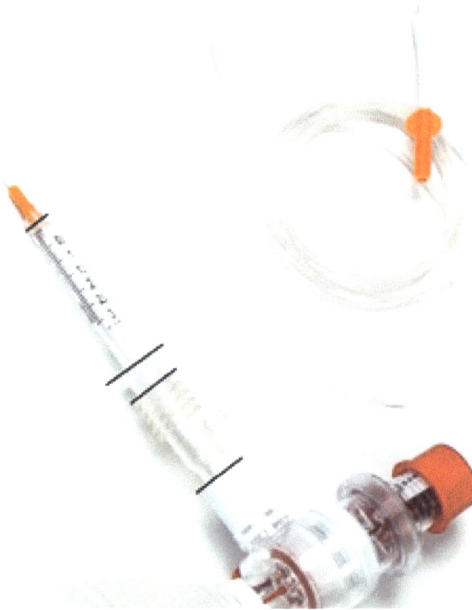

*Needle cricothyrotomy will not fully ventilate the patient, but it can allow for introduction of small amounts of oxygen to reduce severity of hypoxia

Questions:

1. You and your partner launch on a scene flight to rendezvous with a ground crew and arrive on scene to find a 5-year-old child in respiratory failure and the ground crew panicked. They tell you that they have tried to intubate twice without success and the child's O$_2$ sats are 71%. What is your priority intervention?

   a) DSI
   b) Provide assisted ventilations
   c) Start an IV
   d) Needle cricothyrotomy

2. While looking at a chest x-ray of an intubated patient, you verify the endotracheal tube insertion depth. Which of the following below identifies the correct depth of an ETT?

   a) 4 in above the carina
   b) At the level of the carina
   c) At the level of T3
   d) Waveform capnography

3. You have placed an endotracheal tube using video laryngoscopy while on scene of an MVC. You and your partner both visualized the tube pass through the vocal cords. What additional confirmation is required?

   a) None, the visualization of the tube passing through cords is sufficient
   b) Chest x-ray
   c) Waveform capnography
   d) SpO_2 >92%

4. When attempting to intubate a patient pulled from a house fire, there is no chest rise with bag valve mask ventilations using proper technique and the patient's SpO_2 is 64%. The patient is unresponsive and apneic, but has a strong, rapid pulse. You should:

   a) Prepare for RSI
   b) Attempt immediate intubation without medications
   c) Administer epinephrine
   d) Surgical cricothyrotomy

Chapter 1 citations:

1. Wolfe, A., Santiago, J., Frakes, M., & Farmer, S. (2022). Critical Care Transport Core Curriculum (2nd ed.). Jones and Bartlett Learning.

2. Mejia, A. (2022). Critical Care Transport (3rd ed.). Jones and Bartlett Learning.

3. Nausheen, F., Niknafs, N.P., MacLean, D.J. et al. The HEAVEN criteria predict laryngoscopic view and intubation success for both direct and video laryngoscopy: a cohort analysis. Scand J Trauma Resusc Emerg Med 27, 50 (2019). https://doi.org/10.1186/s13049-019-0614-6

4. Sharma S, Danckers M, Sanghavi D, et al. High Flow Nasal Cannula. [Updated 2022 Sep 21]. In: StatPearls [Internet]. Treasure Island (FL): StatPearls Publishing; 2022 Jan-. Available from: https://www.ncbi.nlm.nih.gov/books/NBK526071/

5. Sole, M. L., Su, X., Talbert, S., Penoyer, D. A., Kalita, S., Jimenez, E., Ludy, J. E., & Bennett, M. (2011). Evaluation of an intervention to maintain endotracheal tube cuff pressure within therapeutic range. American journal of critical care : an official publication, American Association of Critical-Care Nurses, 20(2), 109–118. https://doi.org/10.4037/ajcc2011661

6. Ahmed RA, Boyer TJ. Endotracheal Tube. [Updated 2022 Aug 9]. In: StatPearls [Internet]. Treasure Island (FL): StatPearls Publishing; 2022 Jan-. Available from: https://www.ncbi.nlm.nih.gov/books/NBK539747/

7. Caroline, N. L. & American Academy of Orthopaedic Surgeons (AAOS). (2017). Nancy Caroline's Emergency Care in the Streets (8th ed.). Jones & Bartlett Learning.

Chapter 2: Arterial blood gas interpretation

What information is on an ABG?
pH
$PaCO_2$
HCO_3
BE
PaO_2
SaO_2
Hemoglobin
Carboxyhemoglobin
Lactate
Potassium
Glucose

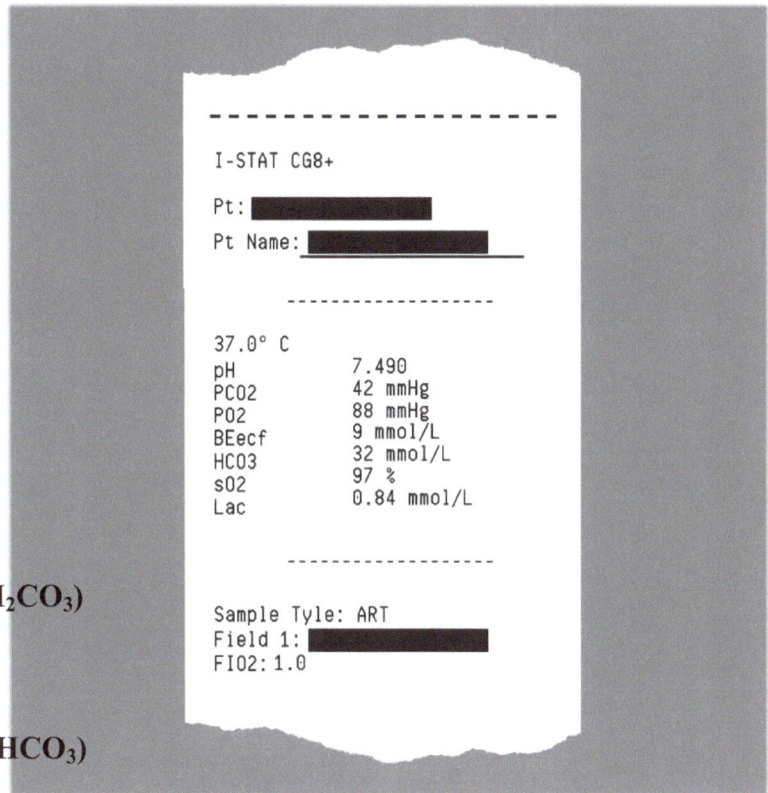

Acid Base Buffering System

Bicarb (HCO_3) and Carbonic Acid (H_2CO_3)
- **Affects pH in seconds**

Lungs blow off/hold CO_2
- **Affects pH in minutes**

Kidneys resorb/excrete bicarbonate (HCO_3)
- **Affects pH in hours to days**

```
  - - - - - - - - - - - - - - - - -

  I-STAT CG8+

  Pt: ████████████████

  Pt Name: ██████████████
           _____

  - - - - - - - - - - - - - -

  37.0° C
  pH          7.490
  PCO2        42 mmHg
  PO2         88 mmHg
  BEecf       9 mmol/L
  HCO3        32 mmol/L
  sO2         97 %
  Lac         0.84 mmol/L

  - - - - - - - - - - - - - -

  Sample Tyle: ART
  Field 1: ██████████████
  FIO2: 1.0
```

Arterial pH 7.35-7.45

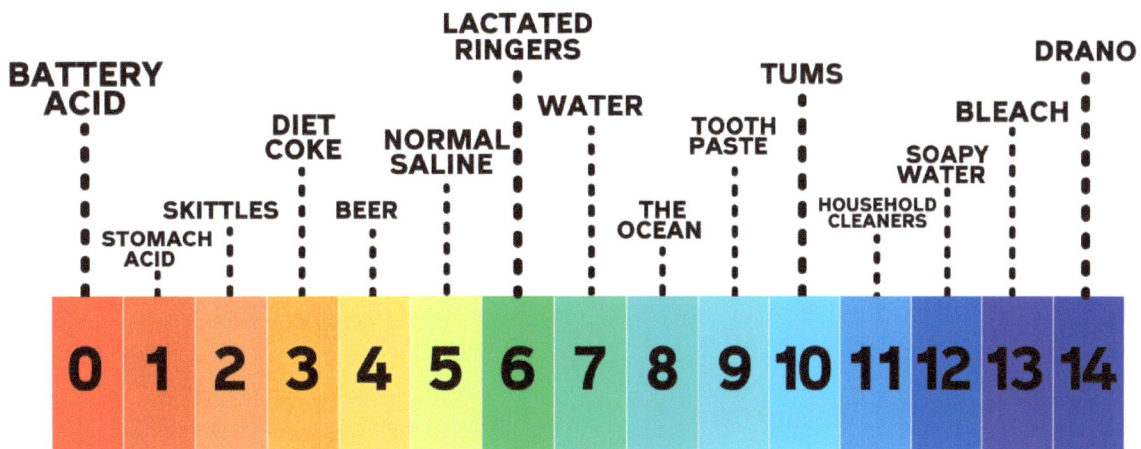

pH

<7.35	7.35-7.45	>7.45
Acidosis	Normal	**Alkalosis**

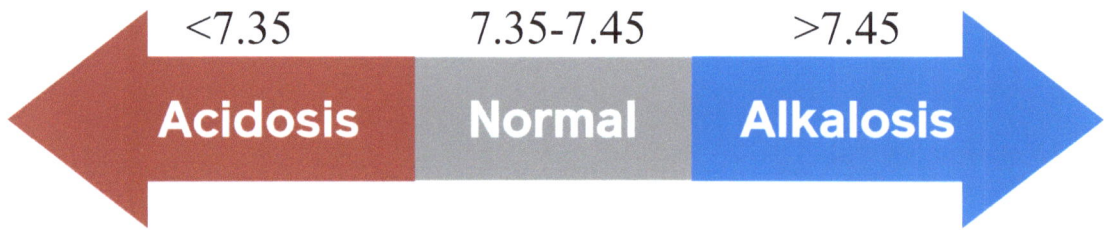

Carbon Dioxide (CO_2)
CO_2 indicates acid, is a waste product of cellular metabolism

- **Expressed in partial pressures ($PaCO_2$)**

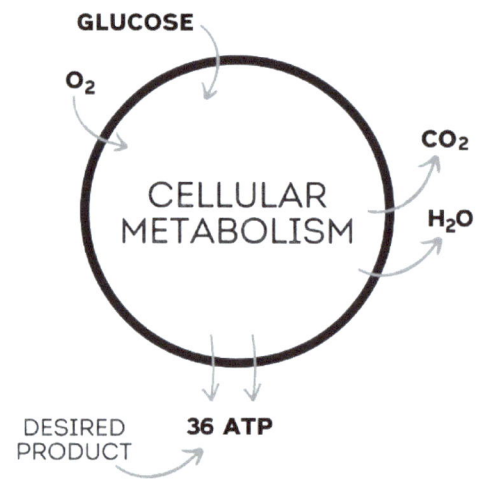

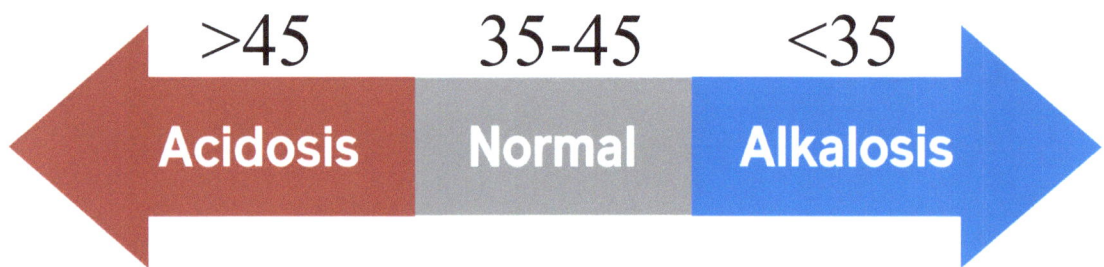

>45	35-45	<35
Acidosis	Normal	Alkalosis

Bicarbonate (HCO_3)

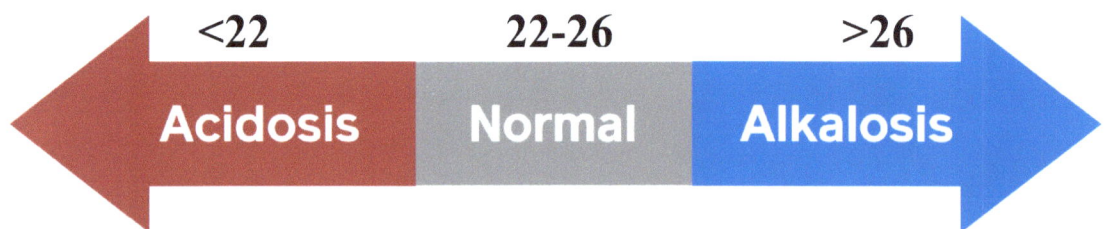

<22	22-26	>26
Acidosis	**Normal**	**Alkalosis**

Base Excess | Base Deficit (BE)
- **Normal: -3 to 3 mEq/L**
- **Positive integer= base excess**
- **Negative integer= base deficit**
- **Indicator of acidosis**

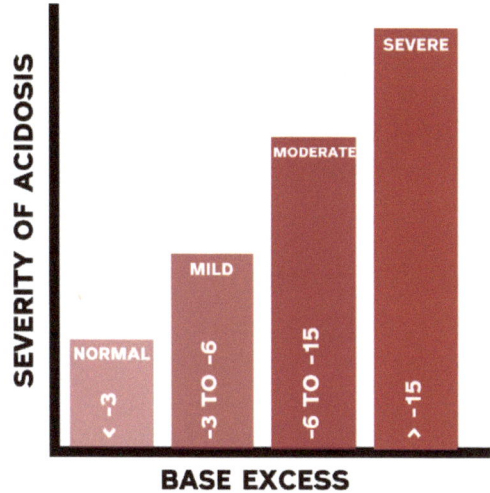

Oxygenation Status
- **PaO$_2$ | Normal 80-100 mmHg**
  - **Plasma concentration of dissolved oxygen**
- **SaO$_2$ | Normal 92-98%**
  - **Percent of hemoglobin bound with oxygen**

40 MMHG **= 70** % SPO2
SEVERE HYPOXEMIA - IMMEDIATE INTERVENTION

50 MMHG **= 80** % SPO2
HYPOXEMIA - NEEDS SUPPLEMENTAL OXYGEN

60 MMHG **= 90** % SPO2
NORMAL - NO INTERVENTIONS NEEDED

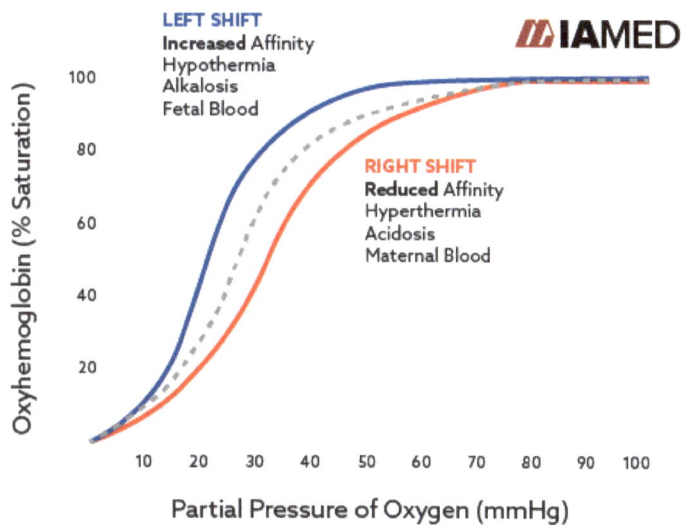

Oxyhemoglobin Dissociation Curve

LEFT SHIFT
Increased Affinity
Hypothermia
Alkalosis
Fetal Blood

RIGHT SHIFT
Reduced Affinity
Hyperthermia
Acidosis
Maternal Blood

Oxyhemoglobin (% Saturation)

Partial Pressure of Oxygen (mmHg)

Interpreting ABGs

Step 1: pH HIGH/LOW/NORMAL?
- **High: Alkalosis**
- **Low: Acidosis**

Step 2: CO2 HIGH/LOW/NORMAL?
- **High: Acidosis**
- **Low: Alkalosis**

Step 3: HCO3 HIGH/LOW/NORMAL?
- **High: Alkalosis**
- **Low: Acidosis**

Step 4: Collate the previous three elements
- If CO_2 is responsible for pH derangement, it is respiratory
- If HCO_3 is responsible for pH derangement, it is metabolic

```
I-STAT CG8+
Pt: ██████████████
Pt Name:_____

------------------
37.0° C
pH              7.490
PCO2            42 mmHg
PO2             88 mmHg
BEecf           9 mmol/L
HCO3            32 mmol/L
sO2             97 %
Lac             0.84 mmol/L
------------------
Sample Tyle: ART
Field 1:██████████████
FIO2: 1.0
------------------
```

pH: Alkalosis

CO_2: Normal

HCO_3: Alkalosis

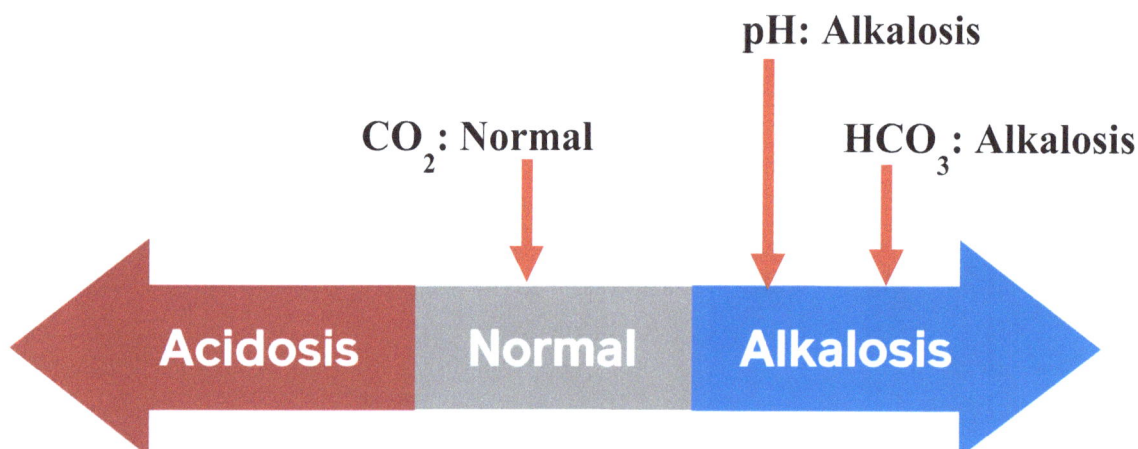

Acidosis   Normal   Alkalosis

Step 5: Compensation
- **Did the non-offending component attempt to correct the pH?**
- **Full compensation: brought pH back into normal range 7.35-7.45**
- **Partial compensation: did not fully correct pH**

Correct Answer of above ABG:
- **Uncompensated Metabolic Alkalosis**

Practice ABGs

1.

```
- - - - - - - - - - - - - - - - - - -
I-STAT CG8+
Pt: ██████████████████
Pt Name:_____

        - - - - - - - - - - - - - - - - - -
37.0° C
pH          7.200
PCO2        60 mmHg
PO2         65 mmHg
BEecf       6 mmol/L
HCO3        25 mmol/L
sO2         98 %
Lac         2.57 mmol/L
        - - - - - - - - - - - - - - - - - -
Sample Tyle: ART
Field 1:███████████████
FIO2: 1.0
- - - - - - - - - - - - - - - - - - -
```

2.

```
- - - - - - - - - - - - - - - - - - -
I-STAT CG8+
Pt: ██████████████████
Pt Name:_____

        - - - - - - - - - - - - - - - - - -
37.0° C
pH          7.258
PCO2        39 mmHg
PO2         90 mmHg
BEecf       3 mmol/L
HCO3        16 mmol/L
sO2         95 %
Lac         5.98 mmol/L
        - - - - - - - - - - - - - - - - - -
Sample Tyle: ART
Field 1:███████████████
FIO2: 0.40
- - - - - - - - - - - - - - - - - - -
```

3.

```
- - - - - - - - - - - - - - - - -
I-STAT CG8+
Pt: ███████████████
Pt Name:_____

       - - - - - - - - - - - - - -
37.0° C
pH          7.376
PCO2        60 mmHg
PO2         65 mmHg
BEecf       2 mmol/L
HCO3        29 mmol/L
sO2         92 %
Lac         0.76 mmol/L
       - - - - - - - - - - - - -
Sample Tyle: ART
Field 1:███████████████
FIO2: 0.60
- - - - - - - - - - - - - - - - -
```

4.

```
- - - - - - - - - - - - - - - - -
I-STAT CG8+
Pt: ███████████████
Pt Name:_____

       - - - - - - - - - - - - - -
37.0° C
pH          7.297
PCO2        68 mmHg
PO2         49 mmHg
BEecf       4 mmol/L
HCO3        32 mmol/L
sO2         99 %
Lac         9 mmol/L
       - - - - - - - - - - - - -
Sample Tyle: ART
Field 1:███████████████
FIO2: 1.00
- - - - - - - - - - - - - - - - -
```

Metabolic Disturbances

Metabolic Alkalosis: pH >7.45, HCO_3 >26
- Often occurs with accumulation of bases or loss of acids and electrolyte imbalances
- Vomiting or gastric suctioning
- Potassium loss due to diuretic use, steroid use, diarrhea
- Antacid overuse
- Treatment:
    - Identify and treat underlying cause
    - Emergent intervention if HCO_3 >55 or pH >7.55
    - Expect profound dehydration and electrolyte depletion
    - Fluid resuscitation
    - Electrolyte replacement

Metabolic Acidosis: pH <7.35, HCO_3 <22
- Lactic acidosis:
    - Sepsis
    - Anaerobic metabolism
    - Ineffective CO_2 clearance* caused by malperfusion
    *DO NOT CONFUSE THIS WITH respiratory pathologies. This isn't respiratory acidosis because the patient isn't breathing off CO_2, it's because circulation is compromised, and CO_2 isn't being transported back to the lungs for elimination

- Cellular starvation states:
    - DKA
    - Alcoholic keto-acidosis
    - Severe malnutrition
- Prolonged seizures
- Rhabdomyolysis
- Toxic exposure
- Hyperkalemia/fever
- Fluid resuscitation
- Hypotension
- Acidosis (of metabolic OR respiratory origin) causes increase in cellular membrane permeability
- Treatment:
    - Identify and treat underlying cause
    - Anticipate and assess for renal dysfunction

Respiratory Disturbances

Respiratory Alkalosis: pH >7.45, CO_2 <35
- Alveolar hyperventilation
  - Pain
  - Anxiety
  - Pregnancy
  - High altitude
  - Over-bagging patient
  - Pulmonary embolism
- Aspirin overdose
- Treatment:
  - Identify and treat underlying cause
- Decrease minute ventilation
  - Carpopedal spasms

Respiratory Acidosis: pH <7.35, CO_2 >45
- Failure of lungs to eliminate CO_2
  - Hypoventilation/apnea
  - Chest wall injury
  - CNS depression
  - Reactive airway
  - Airway obstruction
  - Cardiac arrest
- Treatment:
  - Identify and treat underlying cause: poor ventilation
- Hypoventilation
  - Obstructive pathology
  - Reactive airway
  - Apnea

Critical ABG Thresholds
- Severe shock
  - pH <7.2
- Hypercarbic respiratory failure
  - CO_2 >55
- Hypoxic respiratory failure
  - PaO_2 <60

Expected Changes

pH & CO_2

- For every change in 10mmHg of $ETCO_2$, the pH will change 0.08 the <u>opposite</u> direction.
- Prior to IFT, a patient's ABG reveals pH 7.20 and CO_2 50. During transport, the crew increases minute ventilation to titrate to $ETCO_2$ 30. What can we expect the pH to be?

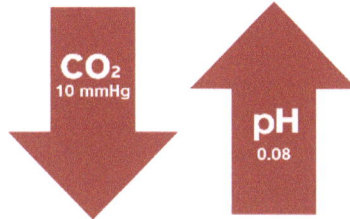

pH & Bicarbonate

- For every change in 0.15 in pH, the HCO_3 will change 10 mmol/L the <u>same</u> direction.
- If the patient's initial ABG revealed a pH of 7.20 and bicarb of 16, but we have corrected the underlying pathology and now have a bicarb of 26, what can we expect the pH to be?

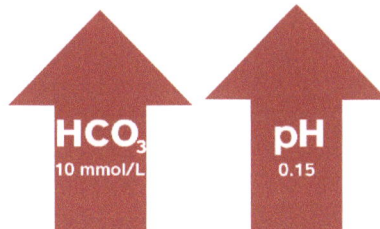

pH & Potassium

- For every change in 0.10 in pH the K^+ will change 0.6 mEqs the <u>opposite</u> direction.
- A patient in metabolic acidosis has a pH of 7.20 and a K^+ of 4.0. After correction of the primary pathology, the pH is now 7.40. What can we expect the K^+ to be now?

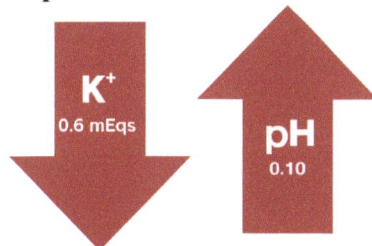

CO$_2$ & Potassium
- For every change in 10 mmHg in CO$_2$ the K$^+$ will change 0.5 mEqs the <u>same</u> direction.
- The patient currently has an ETCO$_2$ of 55 and a serum K$^+$ of 3.5. During transport the ventilator is titrated to ETCO$_2$ of 35. What can we expect the K$^+$ to be?

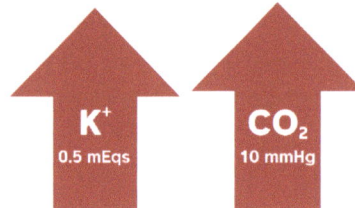

ABG Scenarios

5. 66-year-old female with history of CHF, DM2, and GERD with an allergy to penicillin and shellfish reports feeling "sick." She is alert to self, but believes it is 1962 and that you are her son Wayne, but her neighbor tells you "She's usually sharp as a tack!" You grab her basket of home meds and see that she is on Lasix, Metformin, and there is a nearly empty Tums bottle.

pH 7.5 | CO$_2$ 36 | HCO$_3$ 29 | PaO$_2$ 97 | SaO$_2$ 97% | BE 5

6. A 14-year-old boy is forced to run a mile in PE class and tells his teacher he needs to stop and rest, that he's having a hard time breathing. The PE teacher tells him to toughen up and keep running. The boy collapses at the end of the mile and is restless and repeatedly states "I can't breathe." The school calls 911 and hands you his demographic sheet which states he has a history of ADHD and asthma.

pH 7.30 | CO$_2$ 49 | HCO$_3$ 25 | PaO$_2$ 79 | SaO$_2$ 86% | BE 1

7. A 71-year-old male presents to the ED for mild shortness of breath and reports his "breathing machine broke" so he cannot take his home nebulized treatments. He is speaking in full sentences but has increased work of breathing with ambulation and has an open pack of cigarettes in his shirt pocket.

pH 7.36 | CO$_2$ 50 | HCO$_3$ 29 | PaO$_2$ 91 | SaO$_2$ 89% | BE 3

Chapter 3: Pulmonary Emergencies

Chest X-Ray

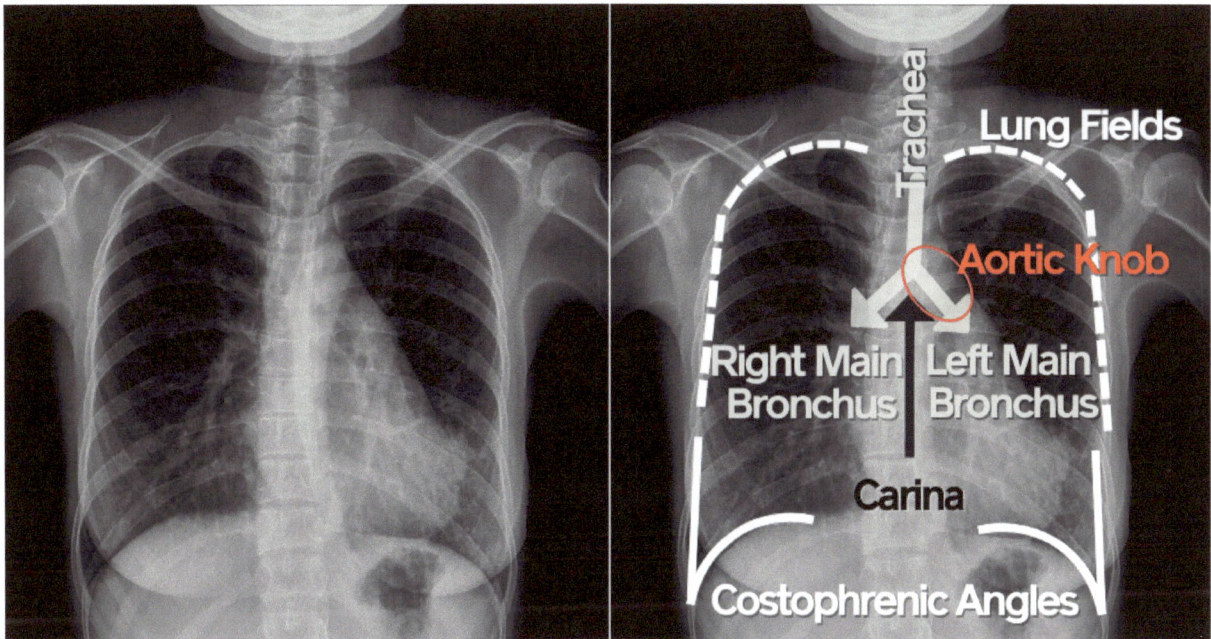

Labels: Trachea, Lung Fields, Aortic Knob, Right Main Bronchus, Left Main Bronchus, Carina, Costophrenic Angles

Components of Oxygenation

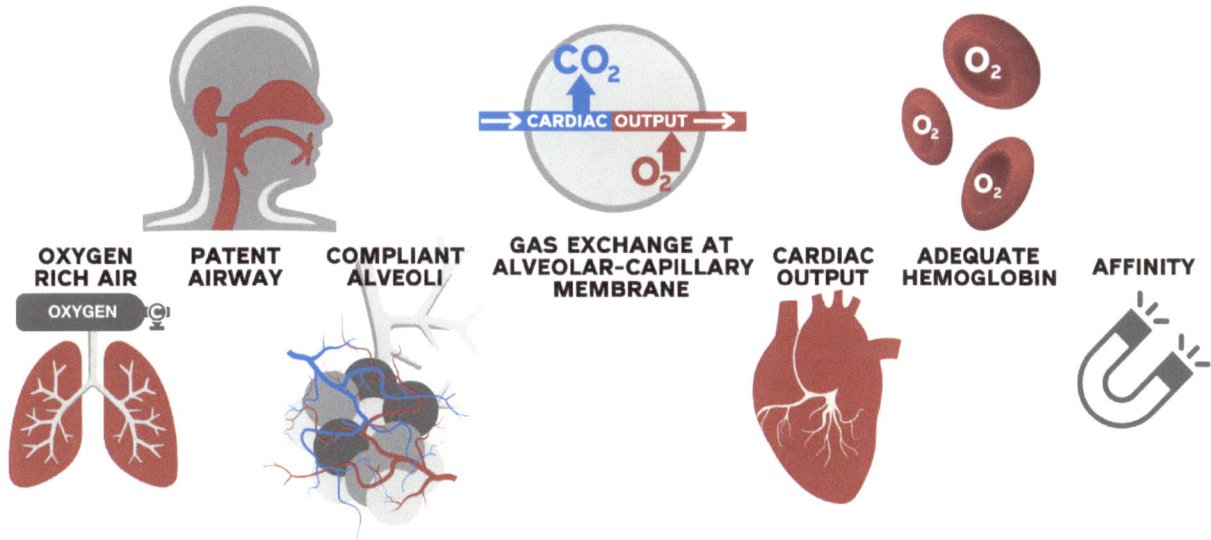

OXYGEN RICH AIR — OXYGEN

PATENT AIRWAY

COMPLIANT ALVEOLI

GAS EXCHANGE AT ALVEOLAR-CAPILLARY MEMBRANE — CO_2, CARDIAC OUTPUT, O_2

CARDIAC OUTPUT

ADEQUATE HEMOGLOBIN — O_2

AFFINITY

Restrictive Conditions

Pulmonary Edema[4,5]
- **Plasma shifts from vasculature to lung parenchyma**
  - **Cardiogenic**
  - **Non-cardiogenic**
- **Symptoms: dyspnea, anxiety, pink frothy sputum**
- **Treatment: NIV, antihypertensives**

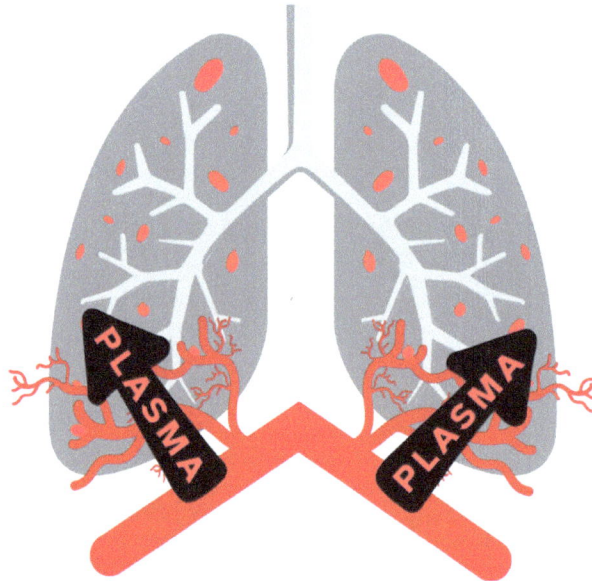

Pleural effusion[4]
- **Collection of fluid between pleural layers**
  - **Maintain high Fowler position**
  - **Supplemental oxygen**
  - **Thoracentesis**

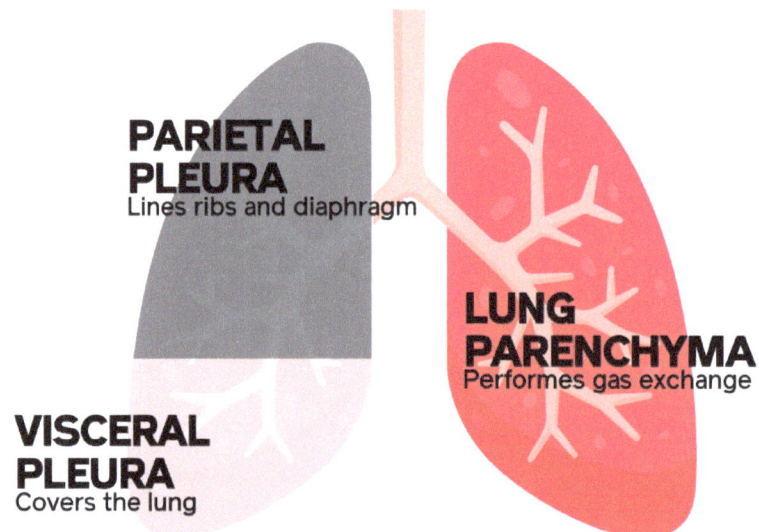

PARIETAL PLEURA
Lines ribs and diaphragm

LUNG PARENCHYMA
Performes gas exchange

VISCERAL PLEURA
Covers the lung

Acute Respiratory Distress Syndrome (ARDS)[3]
- Occurs in response to primary injury or illness
  - Sepsis
  - Pancreatitis
  - Hypovolemic shock
  - Pulmonary contusion
  - Burns
- High risk for ventilator associated injury
- ARDS assessment findings
  - Precipitating insult
  - Hypoxia
  - Dyspnea if not intubated
  - High ventilator pressures if mechanically ventilated
  - Pulmonary edema
  - Ground glass chest radiography appearance

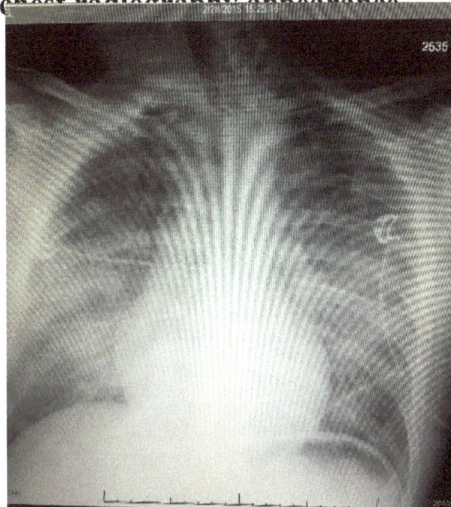

P:F Ratio
- Quick tool to look at severity of ARDS
- Not accurate in patients with VQ mismatch

A comparison of
PaO_2 to FiO_2

Normal: 400+

Mild ARDS: 200-300

Moderate ARDS: 100-200

Severe ARDS: <100

Treatment of ARDS
- Treat underlying cause
- Optimize oxygenation through safe ventilation
  - ARDSnet mechanical ventilation protocol
  - Prone position
  - Maintain alveolar recruitment
- ECMO

Neuromuscular Disease/Injury

- **Muscular dysfunction can lead to decreased efficacy of the diaphragm and chest wall**
  - **Amyotrophic Lateral Sclerosis (Lou Gehrig's Disease)**
  - **Polio**
  - **Myasthenia gravis**
  - **Guillain Barre**
  - **Spinal cord injuries**

Pneumonia[3]

- **Inflammatory process affecting lower airway**
  - **Intrapulmonary shunt**
- **Offending pathogen**
  - **Viral**
  - **Fungal**
  - **Bacterial**
  - **Parasitic**
- **Symptoms:**
  - **Hypoxemia, productive cough, dyspnea, fever, pleuritic chest pain, subjective abdominal fullness, infiltrates on CXR**

Pneumothorax[3]

- **Accumulation of air in pleural space**
  - **Traumatic**
  - **Spontaneous**
- **Symptoms:**
  - **Dyspnea, impending doom, chest pain**
- **If left untreated: tension pneumothorax**
  - **Tracheal deviation**
- **Treatment:**
  - **Simple: observation, O_2 administration**
  - **Severe: decompression, chest tube placement (see below)**
  - **Protect from effects of altitude**

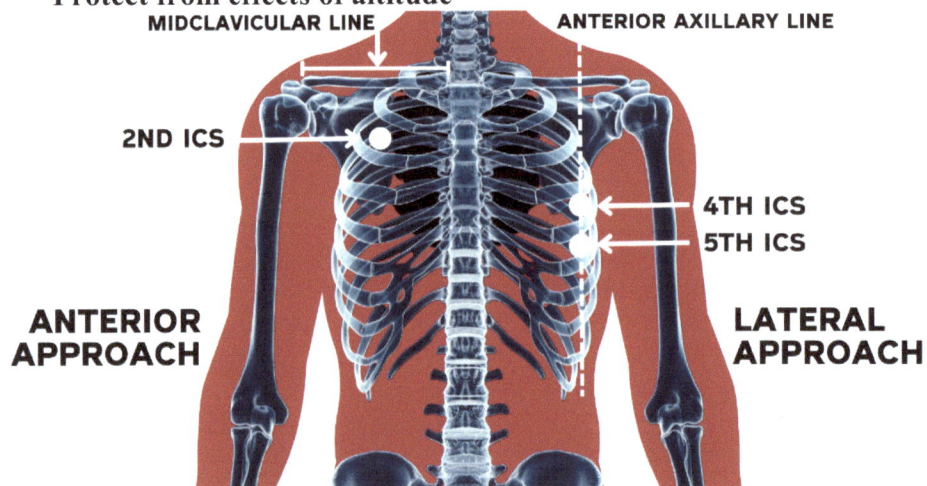

MIDCLAVICULAR LINE   ANTERIOR AXILLARY LINE

2ND ICS

4TH ICS
5TH ICS

ANTERIOR APPROACH   LATERAL APPROACH

Pulmonary Fibrosis[5]

- **Progressive scarring of the lungs**
  - **Supplementary oxygen**
  - **Lung transplant**
  - **Causes: medications, occupational exposure, auto-immune disease, radiation**

Obstructive Conditions

Asthma
- **Inflammation of bronchial walls**
- **Excessive mucus production**
- **Symptoms: wheezes, dyspnea, shortness of air, grunting, orthopnea, fatigue, hypercapnia**
- **Signs of failure in asthma patient**
  - **Absent breath sounds**
  - **Altered mental status**
  - **PaO_2 <60mmHg**
- **Treatment: remove trigger, beta-2 agonists, bronchodilators, steroids, ventilatory support, extend expiratory time, ZEEP**

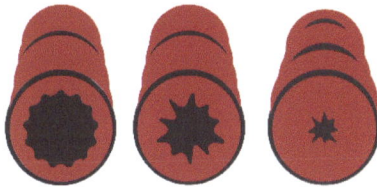

Bronchoconstriction

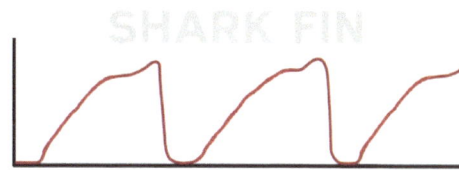

ECTO$_2$ waveform

Chronic Obstructive Pulmonary Disease (COPD)[4,5]

Emphysema: damage to ends of bronchioles, alveoli merge into bullae
- **Barrel chest, tachypnea,**
- **Chronic lung hyperinflation caused by increased airway resistance and decreased elastic recoil**
- **"Pink puffer"**

Chronic bronchitis: excessive mucus production in bronchial tree
- **Productive cough, rhonchi, hypercapnia, hypoxemia, cor pulmonale**
- **"Blue bloater"**

COPD Treatment:
- **Non-invasive ventilation**
  - **Start at PIP 10 cmH$_2$O and PEEP 5 cmH$_2$O**
- **Bronchodilators**
- **Corticosteroids**
- **Antibiotics**
- **If intubated:**
  - **Extended expiratory time (1:4+)**
  - **Low rate (10-12)**

- **Set PEEP at 75% less than the patient's auto-PEEP**

V/Q Mismatch

Ventilation(V)/Perfusion(Q) Ratio[5]
- **Inadequate ventilation or perfusion**
- **V/Q mismatch**
  - **Ventilation disruption: "shunt"**
  - **Perfusion disruption: "dead space ventilation"**

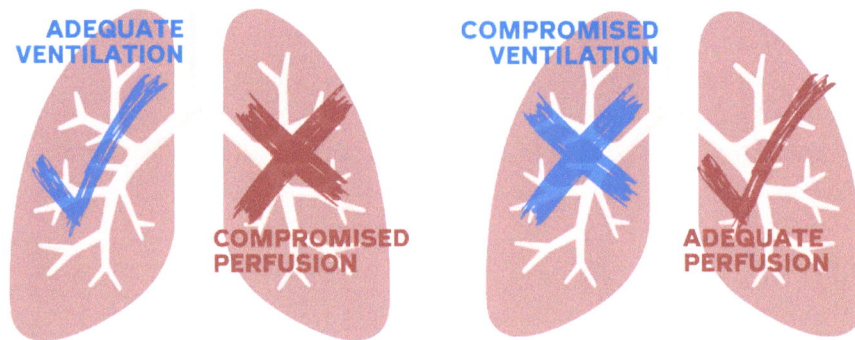

Aa Gradient
Normal: 10-15 mmHg

$$P_AO_2 = FiO_2 \times (P_{atm} - P_{H_2O}) - \frac{P_aCO_2}{RQ}$$

V/Q: Sickle cell anemia acute chest
- **Sickle-shaped red blood cells that clump and form vaso-occlusions**
  - **Extreme pain**
  - **Anemia**
  - **Weakness/fatigue**
- **Acute chest syndrome**
- **Treatment: hydration, oxygen therapies, blood transfusion, pain management**

Pulmonary Embolism[1]

- **Obstruction in pulmonary artery**
  - **Acute: symptoms develop immediately**
  - **Subacute: symptoms present days/weeks later**
  - **Chronic: slow development of pulmonary hypertension over many years**

PE Risk Factors[1]

- **Pregnancy**
- **Malignancy**
- **Stroke**
- **Recent surgery**
- **Traumatic SCI**
- **Recent orthopedic procedures**
- **Oral birth control use**
- **Inherited thrombotic disorders**
- **Nephrotic syndrome: causes coagulation disorders**

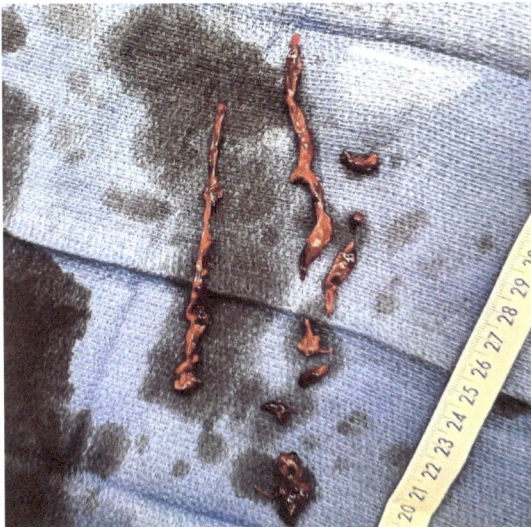

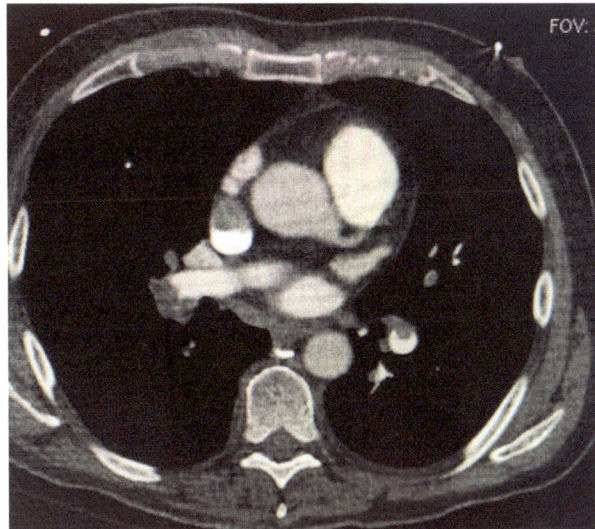

Massive vs. Sub-massive PE[1]

- **Massive indicates hemodynamically instability**
- **Sub-massive presents with associated RV strain**
- **Low-risk PE has no evidence of RV strain**

PE Treatment[1,2]

- **May require thrombolysis**
- **HFNC and pulmonary vasodilators**
- **Mainstay treatment remains heparin and anticoagulation**
- **May have surgical clot removal in extreme cases**
- **DO NOT over-administer fluids**

Septic Emboli
- **Many micro-emboli caused by infectious process, often associated with IVDU and endocarditis**

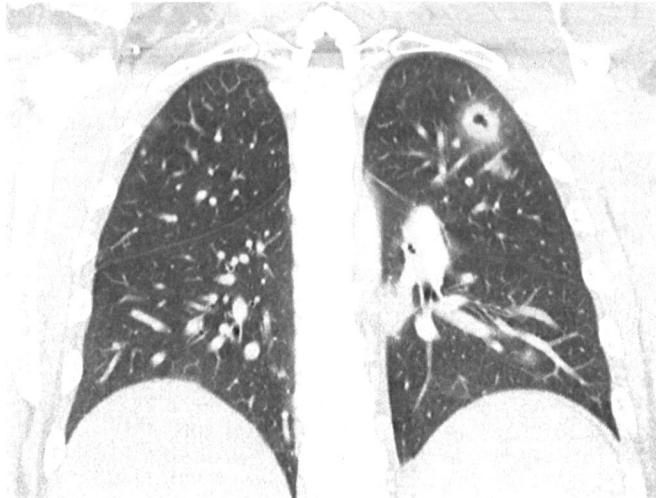

Respiratory Failure

Acute respiratory failure[3]
- **PaO_2 <60mmHg on room air**
- **SpO_2 <90%**
- **$PaCO_2$ >50mmHg**
- **Causes: CNS depression, altitude, chest wall injury, toxic exposure, exacerbation of chronic lung disease, infection**

Hypoxic Respiratory Failure
- **PaO_2 <60mmHg on room air**
- **SpO_2 <90%**
- **Inadequate delivery of oxygen to tissues**
- **Identify and treat primary cause of respiratory failure**

Hypercapnic Respiratory Failure
- **$PaCO_2$ >50mmHg**
- **Inadequate ventilation, elimination of CO_2**
- **Identify and treat primary cause of respiratory failure**

questions:

1. You and your partner rendezvous with a BLS ground crew for a 49-year-old female whose husband called 911 when she tried to get up to the restroom in the night and collapsed. She is cyanotic, tachypneic, and keeps saying "I'm going to die!" The husband tells you her only medical history is uterine fibroids, which she just had a hysterectomy for 5 days ago.

   What's your differential and what is your plan?

2. A patient with cardiogenic pulmonary edema is being transported via long-distance, high- altitude, fixed-wing transport. The patient's respiratory status has deteriorated; the patient is dyspneic, mildly hypoxic, and hypertensive. What is the appropriate plan of action?

   a. BiPAP 6/3 and 20mg IV hydralazine
   b. BiPAP 10/5, IV nitro drip, 40mg IV furosemide
   c. 15L O_2 NRB, IV nitro bolus Q5min
   d. CPAP 40, IV magnesium drip

3. A patient's mother calls 911 for her 14-year-old child experiencing an asthma exacerbation. On auscultation, lung sounds are very quiet in all fields. The flight paramedic places the patient on the monitor and the NIBP reads 88/54. What is the likely cause?

   a. Monitor error due to ill-fitting cuff
   b. Sepsis secondary to pneumonia
   c. Albuterol overdose
   d. Hyperinflated lungs

Chapter 3 Citations:

1) Tubaro, M., Vranckx, P., Price, S., Vrints, C., & Bonnefoy, E. (2021). The ESC Textbook of Intensive and Acute Cardiovascular Care (The European Society of Cardiology Series) (3rd ed.). Oxford University Press.
2) EMCrit, A., & Farkas, J. (2021, November 29). Submassive & Massive PE. EMCrit Project. https://emcrit.org/ibcc/pe/
3) Wolfe, A., Santiago, J., Frakes, M., & Farmer, S. (2022). Critical Care Transport Core Curriculum (2nd ed.). Jones and Bartlett Learning.
4) Caroline, N. L. & American Academy of Orthopaedic Surgeons (AAOS). (2017). Nancy Caroline's Emergency Care in the Streets (8th ed.). Jones & Bartlett Learning.
5) Mejia, A. (2022). Critical Care Transport (3rd ed.). Jones and Bartlett Learning.

Chapter 4: Ventilator management

Respiratory Anatomy

Upper Airway:
- **Nose**
- **Mouth**
- **Pharynx**

Lower Airway:
- **Larynx**
- **Trachea**
- **Bronchus/Bronchioles**
- **Alveoli**

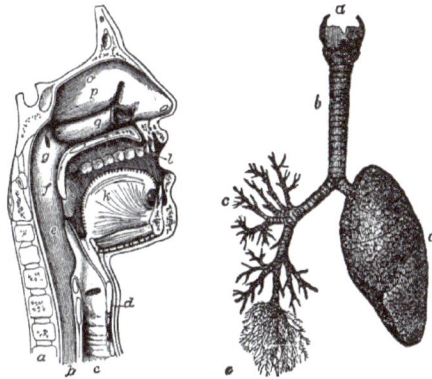

Chemoreceptors
- **Central:**
    - **Medulla/pons**
- **Peripheral:**
    - **Carotid artery and aortic arch**
    - **Response driven by:**
    - **O_2**
    - **CO_2**
    - **H+ levels**

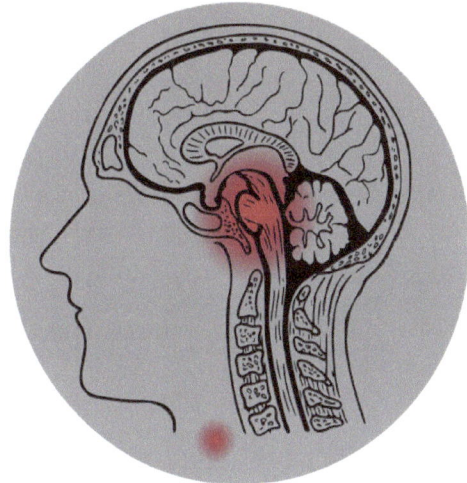

Ventilation vs. Oxygenation
- **Ventilation:**
    - **Movement of air in and out of the lungs**

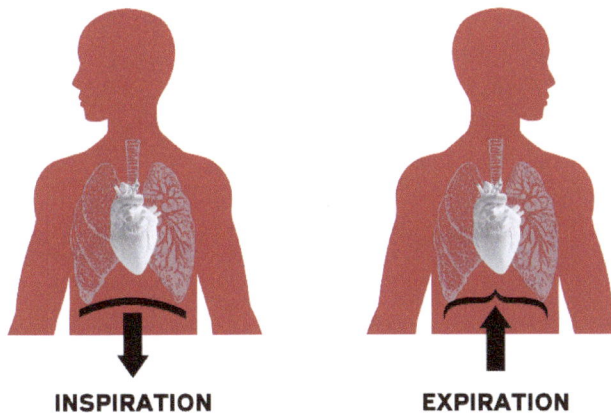

- Oxygenation:
  - Delivery of oxygen to the tissue

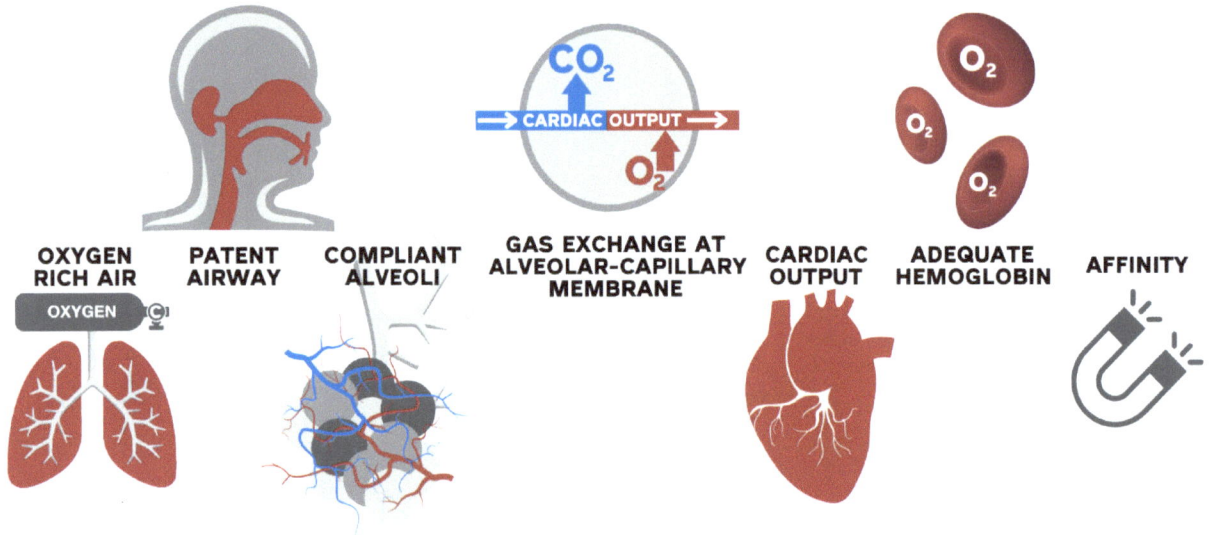

Lung Dynamics

Compliance: Stretchability
- Determines the relationship between volume and pressure when ventilating

$$\frac{V_T}{DRIVING\ PRESSURE} = COMPLIANCE$$

0.1-0.4 L/cmH₂O

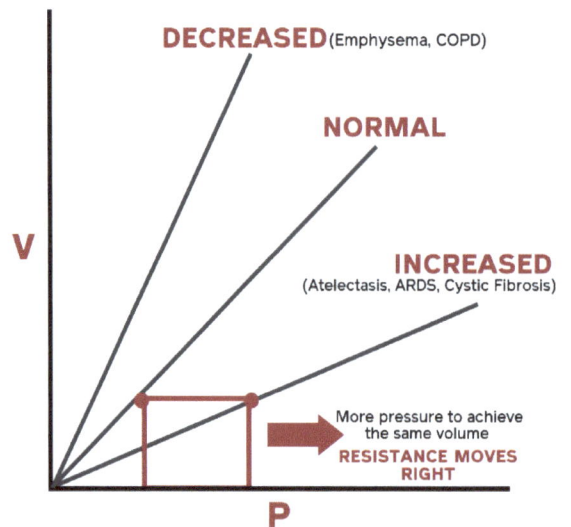

Resistance

48

- **Changes in pressure are proportional to changes in flow, and changes in resistance are inversely proportional to flow**

Dead Space
- **Section of the patient's respiratory system that does not participate in gas exchange**
  - **Anatomical – larger conducting airways (approx. 150ml)**
  - **Alveolar – areas of alveoli without perfusion**
  - **Mechanical- ventilator circuit, adjuncts**

Ventilation/Perfusion Ratios (V/Q)

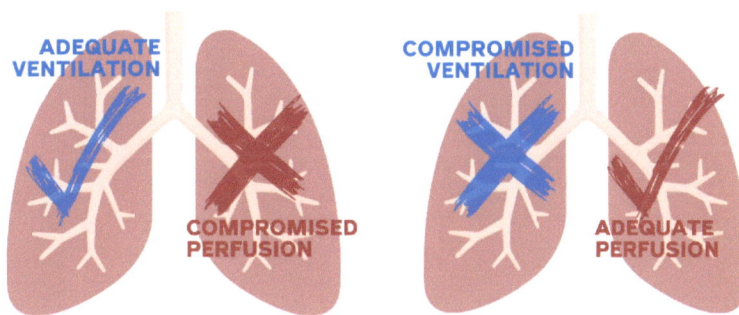

Fick's Law:
- **The rate of diffusion is directly proportional to the difference in partial pressure and the surface area of the membrane. It is inversely proportional to the thickness of the membrane**

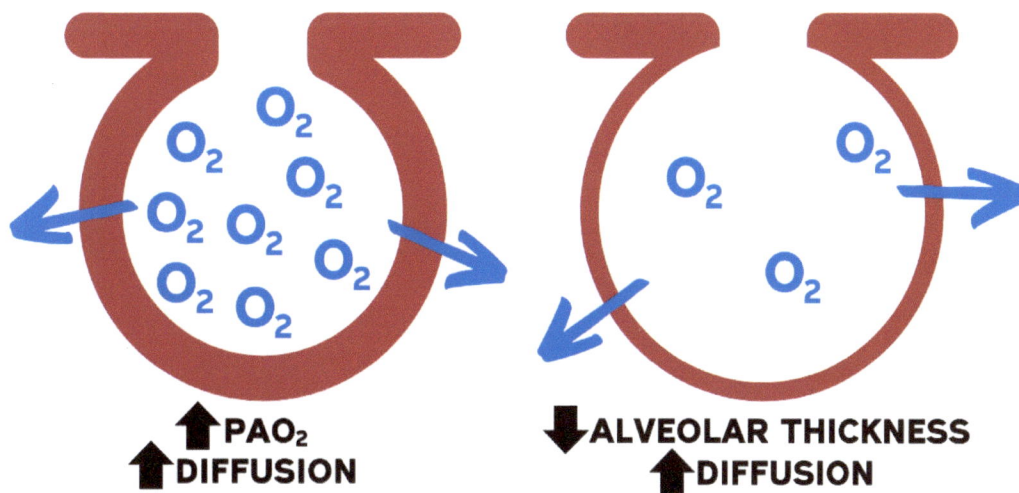

Effects of Mechanical Ventilation

Intra-Thoracic Pressure

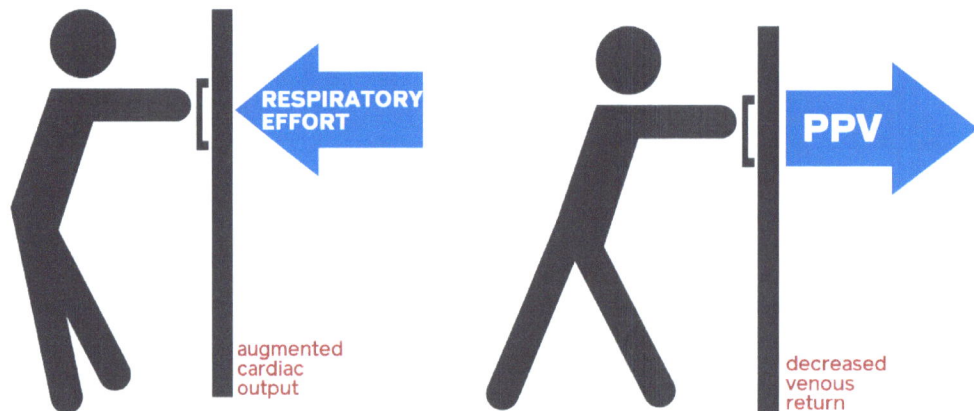

Atelectasis: Collapse of the alveoli
- **Compressive**
- **Cicatricial**
- **Adhesive**
- **Absorptive**
- **Obstructive**

Atelectrauma: Injury to the alveoli cause by constantly opening and closing
- **Repeated alveolar collapse and expansion (RACE)**
- **Driving pressure**

Barotrauma: Injury to the lung caused by pressure
- **Pulmonary interstitial emphysema**
- **Pneumomediastinum**
- **Pneumopericardium**
- **Pneumothorax**
- **Tension pneumothorax**

**Iatrogenic barotrauma is possible with inappropriate ventilator settings

Oxygen Toxicity
- **Release of free radicals**
- **Cerebral vasoconstriction**
- **Can exacerbate absorptive atelectasis**

Ventilator Associated Pneumonia (VAP): Pneumonia that develops in patients within 48 hours after the initiation of ventilation

Long Term Effects

- Stress ulcers
- Malnutrition
- Renal insufficiency
- Neuromuscular effects
- Ventilator dependency
- ICU delirium

How to safely apply A ventilator

Goal of mechanical ventilation:
- Oxygenate
- Ventilate

*Strive to mimic normal physiology as closely as possible

Breath Type: How is your ventilator delivering a breath?
- Pressure control
- Volume control

Modes: Determine how the ventilator will respond to the patient breathing:
- Assist Control
- Synchronized Intermittent Mandatory Ventilation
- Pressure Regulated Volume Control
- Airway Pressure Release Ventilation
- Brand specific modes

Calculating Ideal Body Weight (IBW):
- Adult female: [(# inches >60) x 2.3] + 45.5
- Adult male: [(# inches >60) x 2.3] + 50
- Pediatric:
- Less than 8 years old: IBW = 2 x Age (years) + 9
- Greater than 8 years old: IBW = 3 x Age (years)

Minute Ventilation (V_e)
- Adult: 100ml/kg IBW
- Pediatric: 150mL/kg IBW
- Infant: 200ml/kg IBW

Tidal Volume (V_t)
- Lung protective volumes: 4-8mL/kg IBW
  - 4mL/kg IBW: injured or noncompliant alveoli
  - 6mL/kg IBW: middle of the road, "normal" setting
  - 8mL/kg IBW: targeting increased minute ventilation

Rate (R)
- **Minute ventilation ÷ tidal volume**

Fraction of Inspired Oxygen (FiO$_2$)
- **One of the quickest ways to rapidly improve the patient's oxygenation is to increase the partial pressure of alveolar oxygen by increasing FiO$_2$**

Positive End Expiratory Pressure (PEEP)
- **"The rate of diffusion is proportional to the surface area of the membrane, and it is inversely proportional to the thickness of the membrane."**
- **Physiologic PEEP**
  - **Pediatrics: 3-5 cmH$_2$O**
  - **Adults: 5 cmH$_2$0**
- **Reasons to increase PEEP:**
  - **Hypoxia**
  - **Atelectasis**
  - **Pulmonary edema**
- **Reasons to decrease PEEP:**
  - **Auto-PEEP**

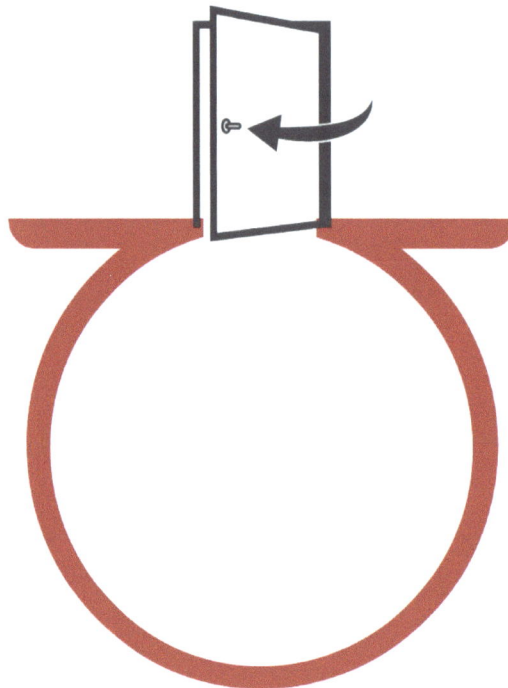

Inspiratory to Expiratory Ratio (I:E)
- Adult 1:2
- Pediatric 1:3
- Infant 1:4

When to adjust:
- Extend e-time: obstructive pathologies
- Extend i-time: non-compliant alveoli
  o 1:1 or inverse ratio

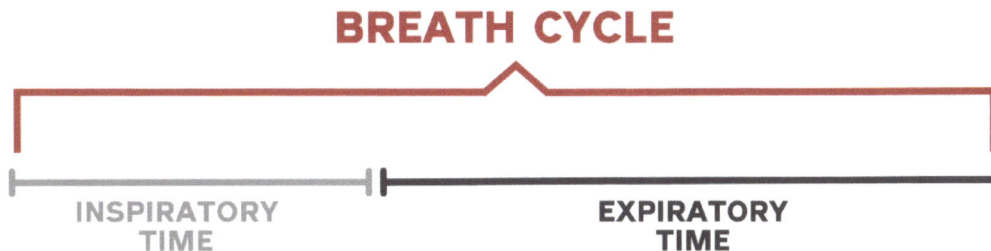

BREATH CYCLE

INSPIRATORY TIME | EXPIRATORY TIME

Peak Inspiratory Pressure (PIP)
- The highest pressure required to deliver the breath (UPPER airway pressure)
  o ETT size
  o Secretions
  o bronchospasm
- Volume: Maximum 35 cmH$_2$O
- Pressure: As low as possible to achieve adequate V_e

Plateau Pressure
- The pressure of a breath dissipated across alveoli (LOWER airway pressure)
- Indicative of alveolar compliance
- Maximum 30 cmH$_2$O
- Driving pressure: P_{plat} – PEEP
  o Goal: less than 15

Rise Time
- Increase when the patient has delicate lungs and the breath needs to be delivered gently
- Short inspiratory rise times are associated with turbulent airflow and increased work of breathing

Pathology Directed Strategies
- **Hypoxic respiratory failure**
  - **Increase PEEP and FiO_2**
- **Hypercarbic respiratory failure**
  - **Increase V_e**
- **Obstructive pathology**
  - **Extend e-time, lengthen breath cycle, ZEEP**
- **Reduced ventilatory drive**
  - **Replace ventilatory drive with "normal" mechanical ventilator settings**

Ventilator Assessment
- **Am I achieving the desired minute ventilation?**
  - **V_e**
  - **V_{te}**
- **Am I within safe pressure parameters?**
  - **PIP**
  - **Pplat**
- **Is my patient Auto-PEEPing?**
- **Vital signs**
- **Patient comfort**

Ventilator Troubleshooting

Oxygenation Issues
- Problem:
  - Lack of adequate oxygen delivery to the tissues
- Identification:
  - SpO_2 monitoring
  - PaO_2
- Solution:
  - FiO_2
  - PEEP

Ventilation Issues
- Problem:
  - Inadequate movement of air in and out of the lungs/alveoli
- Identification:
  - $ETCO_2$ monitoring
  - $PaCO_2$
- Solution:
  - Respiratory Rate
  - Tidal Volume

Ventilator Alarms
- High pressure: obstruction, cough, decreased compliance, circuit kink, increased airway resistance, pneumothorax, dyssynchrony
- Low pressure: dislodged ETT, circuit leak or disconnect, deflated ETT cuff, high spontaneous respiratory drive
- Low V_e: check V_{te} and rate, assess for reasons ventilator is unable to deliver adequate volume

Non-invasive ventilation

CPAP
- Continuous Positive Airway Pressure
  - One pressure throughout duration of breath cycle
  - Best for oxygenation problems & alveolar recruitment
  - Pulmonary edema
  - Pneumonia
  - Neonatal respiratory failure

BiPAP
- Bilevel Positive Airway Pressure
  - Two pressures
    - Inspiratory pressure & Expiratory pressure
  - Best for ventilation problems
    - COPD & asthma

questions:

5'1" female in anaphylactic shock after exposure to peanuts, pre-intubation vitals are:
Pulse 144, NIBP 86/51, RR 55, $EtCO_2$ 26, SpO_2 88% 15L NRB

     IBW

     V_e

     V_t

     Rate

     I:E

     PEEP

     FiO_2

What ventilator assessments should we perform?

6'2" male in an DKA, pre-intubation vitals are:
Pulse 141, NIBP 96/60, RR 46, $EtCO_2$ 11, SpO_2 97%
ABG: pH 6.91, CO_2 10, HCO_3 4

     IBW

     V_e

     V_t

     Rate

     I:E

     PEEP

     FiO_2

What ventilator assessments should we perform?

1. The patient most likely to have immediate complications from endotracheal intubation and mechanical ventilation is:

    a. a patient in DKA
    b. a patient with an acute COPD exacerbation
    c. an asthmatic child
    d. a patient with ARDS secondary to cardiac arrest with ROSC

2. Peak inspiratory pressures above _____ are known to be dangerous to the lungs.

    a. 30 cmH_2O
    b. 45 cmH_2O
    c. 18 cmH_2O
    d. 35 cmH_2O

3. Winter's formula is only applicable in patients with:

a. Respiratory acidosis
b. Metabolic acidosis
c. Respiratory alkalosis
d. Metabolic alkalosis

4. Plateau pressure measures:

a. Highest pressure during the respiratory cycle
b. Alveolar compliance
c. Pressure at the end of the exhalation phase
d. The need for PEEP

Bonus Question: What does a sudden rise in P_{PLAT} indicate?

Chapter 5: Lab Values

Basic Metabolic Panel (BMP)

Na^+ 135-145	Cl^- 96-106	BUN 8-23	Glu 70-110
K^+ 3.5-5.0	HCO_3 22-28	Cr 0.5-1.2	

Sodium[1]
135-145 mEq/L
- Body's primary extracellular ion
- Maintains extracellular fluid volume
- Regulates membrane potential
- Most common electrolyte imbalance

Hypernatremia
- Causes: dehydration, over-diuresis, diabetes insipidus
- Symptoms: tachypnea, sleep disturbances, restlessness
- Treatment: hydration, correction of underlying cause

Hyponatremia
- Causes: SIADH, medications, CHF, overhydration, AKI, excessive sweating
- Symptoms: altered LOC, confusion, seizures if severe
- Treatment: slow hypertonic saline, correction of underlying cause
- Critical low: <120

Potassium
3.5-5.0 mmol/L
- Body's primary intracellular ion
- Responsible for excitability of cardiac membranes
- Is affected by acid-base balance

Hypokalemia
- Causes: diuretic use, n/v/d, renal insufficiency, excessive sweating
- Symptoms: malaise, confusion, paresis, aphasia
- Treatment: Oral potassium (preferred), or IV potassium drip

*Often accompanied by hypomagnesemia

Hyperkalemia

- Causes: medications, renal failure, rhabdomyolysis
- Symptoms: muscle cramps, muscle weakness
- Treatment:
    - Step 1: stabilize cardiac membrane with calcium
    - Step 2: shift potassium into the cell using insulin (must pre-treat with dextrose), bicarbonate (case dependent), and albuterol
    - Step 3: eliminate potassium through dialysis or diuretics

EKG changes associated with hyperkalemia[3]

- Peaked T waves
- PR prolongation
- Widened QRS complex and development of blocks
- Sine wave
- Order of EKG changes as hyperkalemia worsens:

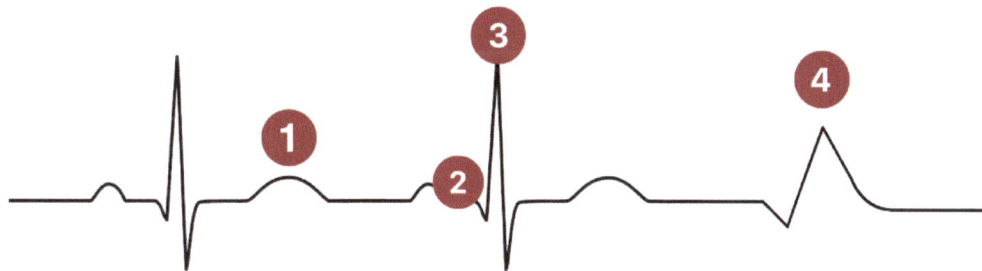

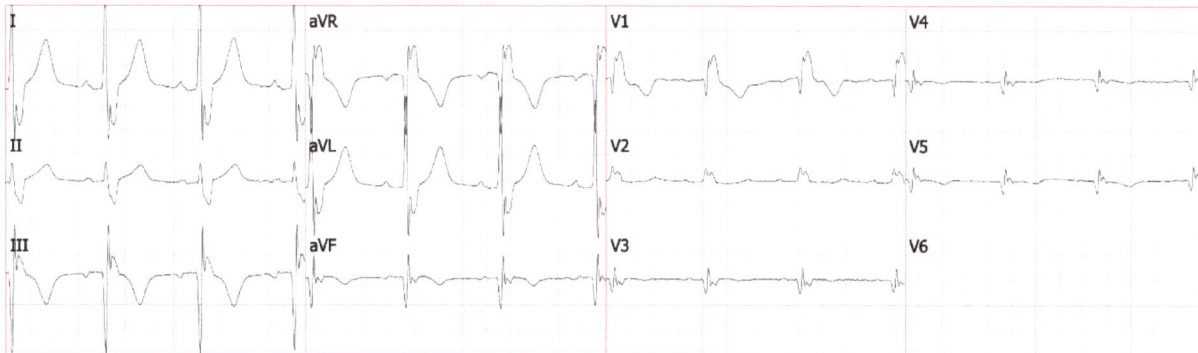

Chloride
96-106 mmol/L

- Hyperchloremia:
    - Causes: over administration of NS or 3% saline, DI
    - Symptoms: fatigue, muscle weakness, excessive thirst, dry mucous membranes
- Hypochloremia: over hydration, SIADH
- Treatments: treat underlying cause

HCO₃/CO₂
22-28 mEq/L

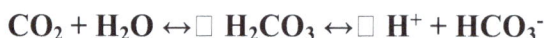

$$CO_2 + H_2O \leftrightarrow H_2CO_3 \leftrightarrow H^+ + HCO_3^-$$

- Indicator of acid-base balance
- Low: metabolic acidosis or respiratory alkalosis
- High: metabolic alkalosis or respiratory acidosis

Anion Gap
8-12 mEq/L

$$Na^+ - (Cl^- + HCO_3^-)$$

- Electrolyte cations minus anions
    - Can be calculated with or without K^+
- Indicator of acidosis

GLYCOLS
ETHYLENE GLYCOL, PROPYLENE GLYCOL

OXOPROLINE
PYROGLUTAMIC ACID, THE TOXIC METABOLITE OF ACETAMINOPHEN

L-LACTATE
LACTIC ACID SEEN IN LACTIC ACIDOSIS

D-LACTATE
EXOGENOUS LACTIC ACID PRODUCED BY GUT BACTERIA

METHANOL
INCLUSIVE OF ALL ALCOHOLS

ASPIRIN
SALICYLATES

RENAL FAILURE
UREMIC ACIDOSIS

KETONES
DIABETIC, STARVATION, ALCOHOLIC

Blood Urea Nitrogen (BUN)
8-23 mg/dL
- Byproduct of protein breakdown
- Elevated levels:
    - Caused by: dehydration, rhabdomyolysis, AKI, chronic renal failure, upper GI bleed
- Treatments: hydration, dialysis, correct underlying issue

Creatinine
0.5-1.2 mg/dL
- Elevated levels: AKI, CKD, rhabdomyolysis
- Treatments: pre-renal, intra-renal, or post-renal?
- Look for trends, where does the patient "live"?

Glucose
70-110 mg/dL
- Hyperglycemia
    - Causes: stress, infection, medications, diabetes
    - Symptoms: altered mental status, polydipsia, polyuria
    - Treatment: rehydration, insulin administration
- Hypoglycemia
    - Causes: inadequate glucose intake, exertion, medications
    - Symptoms: decreased LOC, weakness
    - Treatment: glucose administration

Calcium
8.5-10 mg/dL
- Hypercalcemia
  - Causes: excessive antacid use, endocrine disorders, cancer, medications
  - Symptoms: AMS, fatigue, weakness, nausea, constipation, polyuria
  - EKG changes: Short QT intervals, 1st degree AV block
  - Treatment: correct underlying cause
- Hypocalcemia
  - Causes: decreased calcium intake or malabsorption, increased calcium loss, pancreatitis, endocrine disorders, sepsis, rapid RBC administration
  - Symptoms: AMS, muscle spasms, cardiac dysrhythmias, coagulopathy
  - EKG changes: prolonged QTc
  - Treatment: calcium administration
  - Chvostek Sign: Stimulation of facial nerve leads to facial twitching
  - Trousseau's Sign: Carpopedal spasm of hand and wrist when BP cuff inflated

Magnesium
1.3-2.1 mg/dL
- Second most abundant intracellular cation
- Hypermagnesemia: rare
  - Causes: renal insufficiency, severe dehydration, over administration of magnesium
  - Symptoms: muscle weakness, decreased DTRs, AMS, bradypnea
  - Hypomagnesemia
  - Causes: malabsorption, malnutrition, diarrhea, laxative abuse, pregnancy
  - Symptoms: Torsades de Pointes

Electrolyte Presentations[2]
- Dyspnea: 14.7%
- Confusion: 14%
- Fever: 13.7%
- Edema: 10%
- Rales: 9%
- Normal Sinus Rhythm: 62%
- Sinus Tachycardia: 24%
- Atrial Fibrillation: 7%

Complete Blood Count (CBC)

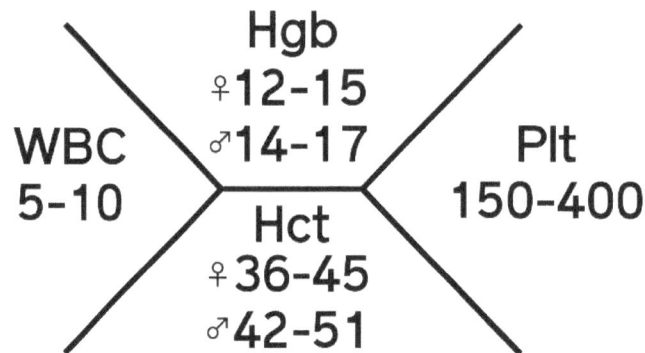

Hgb
♀12-15
♂14-17

WBC
5-10

Plt
150-400

Hct
♀36-45
♂42-51

Hemoglobin
♀ 12-15 g/dL
♂ 14-17 g/dL
- **Elevated levels**
  - **Causes: polycythemia, blood doping, compensation for chronic hypoxia, hemoconcentration**
  - **Treatment: hydration, blood donation**
- **Decreased levels**
  - **Causes: blood loss, anemia, hemolysis, liver dysfunction, SIADH (hemodilution)**
  - **Treatment: PRBC administration, Erythropoetin, treat underlying cause**

Hematocrit
♀ 36-45%
♂ 42-51%
- **A percentage of the blood, by volume, of cellular components, and the remainder is plasma**
- **Should be approximately 3x hemoglobin**

Causes, symptoms, and treatment are similar to deviations in hemoglobin

Blood Transfusion
- **Transfusion should be initiated in the symptomatic actively bleeding patient or hgb <7**
- **Transfuse whole blood or 1:1:1 products**
- **1 PRBC = ↑1 point in hemoglobin and 3% hematocrit**

Blood Transfusion Case Study
- A 49-year-old female weighing 87 pounds presented to ED for increasing weakness. She has markedly yellow skin and conjunctiva. Hgb 1.8, Hct 9%. What's your differential and proposed treatment?
- The physician orders 5 units PRBCs. What should we expect the Hgb and Hct be after transfusion?

White Blood Cell count
5,000-10,000/μL
- Cells mobilized in response to perceived threat to body
- Leukocytosis
  - Caused by: Stress, infection, trauma, extreme exercise, medications, cancer
- Leukocytopenia
  - Caused by: Compromised immune system, medications, cancer, sepsis
  - Protect patient from infection!
  - Treatment: identify and treat underlying cause

Platelets
150,000-400,000/μL
- Thrombocythemia
  - Causes: PE, acute bleeding, metastatic cancer
- Thrombocytopenia
  - Causes: splenomegaly, DIC, cancer or leukemia, sickle cell disease, lupus, chronic liver failure, HIT, ITP
  - Treatments: platelet transfusion
  - Transport considerations: protect from bleeding

Coagulation panel

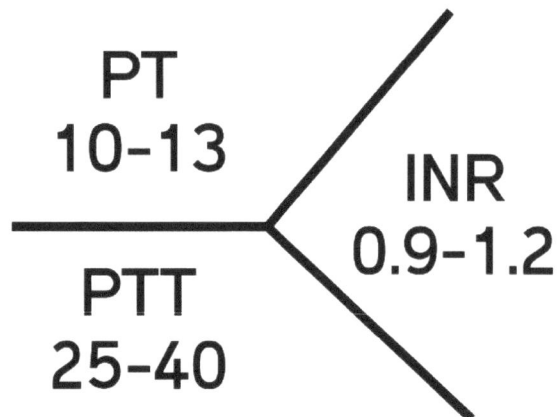

PT
10-13

PTT
25-40

INR
0.9-1.2

International Normalized Ratio[1]
0.8-1.2
- Standard for measuring coagulation status
- Compares patient's PT to control PT
- INR $\geqq$ 5 critical, severe risk for bleeding
- Therapeutic goals:
  - A-fib, history of DVT or PE: 2-3
  - Mechanical mitral valve: 3
  - VAD patients: 4-5

Prothrombin Time
10-13 sec
- Measures how long it takes blood to clot once a reagent is added to it
  - Results vary based on which reagent is used
  - Used to monitor patients on warfarin
- Elevated levels
  - Causes: anticoagulants, liver failure, vitamin K deficiency, DIC, bleeding disorders
  - Symptoms: excessive ecchymosis or bleeding
- Decreased levels
  - Causes: estrogen medications

Reversing Anticoagulants
- Warfarin/Coumadin: Vitamin K
- Heparin and Lovenox: Protamine sulfate
- Eliquis & Xarelto: Kcentra or Andexanet alfa

Liver Panel Values:
- **AST/ALT**
- **Ammonia**
- **Bilirubin**
- **Alkaline Phosphatase**

AST/ALT
AST: 8-48 U/L ALT: 7-55 U/L
- **Elevated levels: indicative of poor liver function**
- **Treatments: treat underlying cause**
- **Transport considerations: be on the lookout for other pathologies associated with liver failure such as ascites (do not lay this patient flat), esophageal varices (do not attempt OG/NG tube insertion), and hepatic encephalopathy**

Ammonia
15-45 µ/dL
- **Hyperammonemia: will cause neurologic changes**
- **Treatments: lactulose**
- **Transport considerations**
  - **Sit up above 30°**
  - **Anti-emetics**
  - **Reduce cerebral edema**

Bilirubin
<1.2 mg/dL
- **Byproduct of RBC breakdown**
- **Elevated levels: often in conjunction with other elevated liver labs**
- **Treatments: treat underlying cause**

Alkaline Phosphatase
30-120 U/L
- **When elevated with AST/ALT, it indicates liver dysfunction**
- **When elevated with bilirubin, it indicates biliary obstruction**
  - **Gallstones**

Amylase and Lipase
Amylase: 30-100 U/L
Lipase: 30-180 U/L
- **Elevated levels: indicates pancreatic pathology, most commonly pancreatitis (300% elevation)**
- **Treatments: treat underlying pathology**
- **Critical thinking: in acute pancreatitis, you will see calcium depletion**

Miscellaneous Values

Lactate
<2 mmol/L
- **Elevated levels**
  - **Causes: anaerobic metabolism secondary to poor perfusion, tissue ischemia**
  - **Treatment: treat underlying cause, fluid bolus**

Troponin[1]
Troponin I <0.4 ng/mL
Troponin T <0.1 ng/mL
- **Released when the heart is overworking**
  - **MI, overexertion, renal failure**

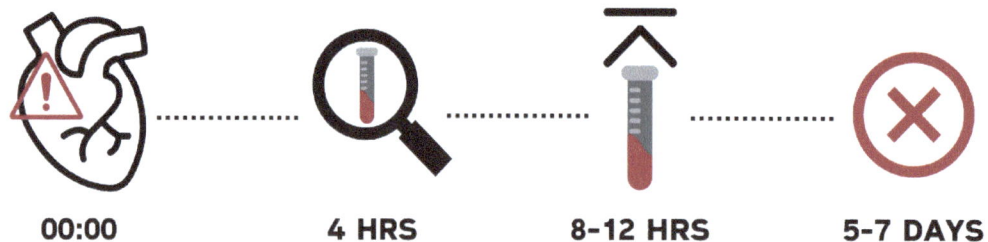

00:00   4 HRS   8-12 HRS   5-7 DAYS

Creatine Kinase[1]
40-150 U/L
- **Released into circulation by damaged muscle, liver, lung, gastrointestinal tissue, kidneys, and spleen when these tissues are damaged**

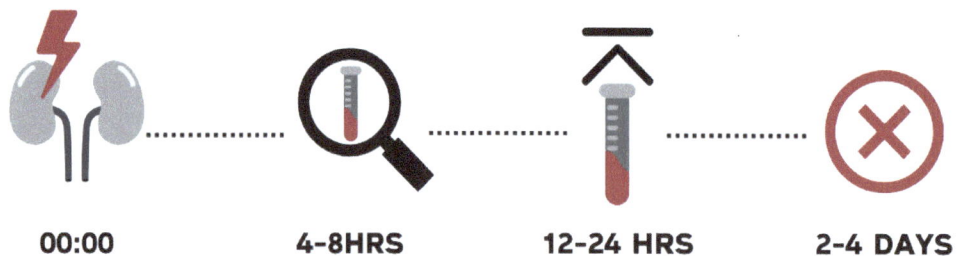

00:00   4-8HRS   12-24 HRS   2-4 DAYS

Inflammatory markers[1]
- **Procalcitonin**
  - **Specific to bacterial infections**
- **C-Reactive Protein**
  - **Non-specific to cause**
- **Erythrocyte Sedimentation Rate**
  - **Non-specific indicator of acute-phase of inflammation**

Chapter 5 Citations:

1. Mejia (Ed.). (2022, April 8). Critical Care Transport (3rd ed.). Jones and Bartlett Learning

2. Colucci, Wilson. (2022). Treatment of Acute Decompensated Heart Failure. Up-to-Date.
3. Caroline, N. L. & American Academy of Orthopaedic Surgeons (AAOS). (2017). Nancy Caroline's Emergency Care in the Streets (8th ed.). Jones & Bartlett Learning.

CHAPTER 6: GENERAL MEDICAL

ENDOCRINE DISORDERS

Diabetes Mellitus[1]
- **Impaired ability to synthesize glucose**
- **Glucose spills into urine**
  - **Three P's Hyperglycemia: Polyuria, Polydipsia, Polyphagia**
- **Prolonged hypoglycemia can cause neuronal damage**

Hyperglycemia[1,7]

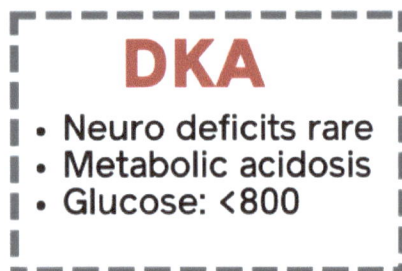

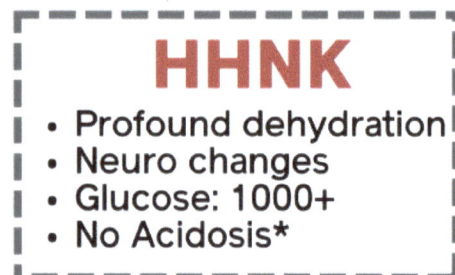

DKA
- Neuro deficits rare
- Metabolic acidosis
- Glucose: <800

HHNK
- Profound dehydration
- Neuro changes
- Glucose: 1000+
- No Acidosis*

SOME FORM OF ACIDOSIS WILL OCCUR DURING CLINICAL COURSE

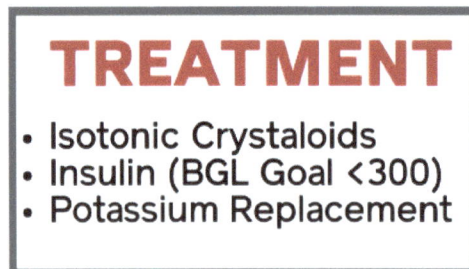

TREATMENT
- Isotonic Crystaloids
- Insulin (BGL Goal <300)
- Potassium Replacement

THYROID DISORDERS

Myxedema Coma[1]
- Low thyroid, results from chronic, untreated hypothyroidism
- Slowed metabolism
- Key presentation triad:
  - Altered mental status, lethargy
  - Thermoregulatory failure
  - Precipitating event

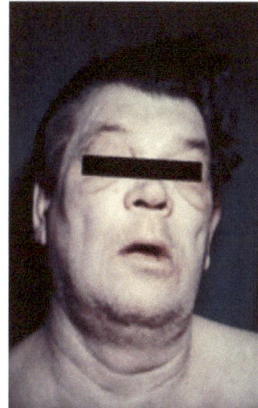

Image: Fred & Van Dijk. http://cnx.org/content/m15004/latest/

Thyroid Storm[5]
- Critical hyperthyroidism
- Known hyperthyroidism with acute changes
- New onset a-fib
- New onset dilated cardiomyopathy
- New onset psychosis w/ abnormal vitals
- Hyperthermia
- CONSIDER IN ANY SEPTIC-APPEARING PATIENT WITHOUT ANY FOCUS OF INFECTION!

ADRENAL DISORDERS

Adrenal Insufficiency[1]
- Addison's Disease
  - Deficiency of steroid hormones, chronic disease
  - Improper regulation of sodium, potassium, and water
- Addisonian crisis
  - Sudden onset exacerbation of Addison's symptoms
  - Shock, AMS, hyperthermia, severe n/v leading to dehydration
  - Can be caused by TBI in patients with no history of Addison's

Cushing's Syndrome
- Too much cortisol production by adrenals
- Weight gain, depression, weakness, thin skin, bruising
- Does not present emergently

Pheochromocytoma
- Catecholamine secreting tumor
  - May present in hypertensive crisis
    - Manage acutely with antihypertensives
  - Requires surgical removal of tumor

PITUITARY DISORDERS

Diabetes Insipidus[9]
- **Insufficient antidiuretic hormone**
  - **Neurogenic: pituitary disorder**
  - **Nephrogenic: poor renal response to ADH**
  - **Dipsogenic: excessive fluid intake**
  - **Gestagenic: rare complication of pregnancy**
- **Huge amounts of dilute urine**
- **Hemoconcentration, hypernatremia**
- **Supportive care, treat primary cause**

SIADH
- **Too much antidiuretic hormone**
  - **Production**
  - **Secretion**
- **Dilutional lab value derangements**
  - **Urine osmolality increases**
  - **Hyponatremia**

ANAPHYLAXIS[18]

CONSIDER ANAPHYLAXIS IN THE PRESENCE OF TWO OR MORE INVOLVED SYSTEMS, EVEN IN THE ABSENCE OF AIRWAY INVOLVEMENT OR HYPOTENSION.
- **Respiratory**
- **Hypotension**
- **Skin Signs**
- **Gastrointestinal**

PRIORITIZE EPINEPHRINE[18]
- **Underutilized**
- **Safe, effective**
  - **Adult dose: 0.3mg IM vastus lateralis**
  - **Pediatric dose: 0.01mg/kg IM vastus lateralis**
- **Deleterious cardiac effects are a myth**

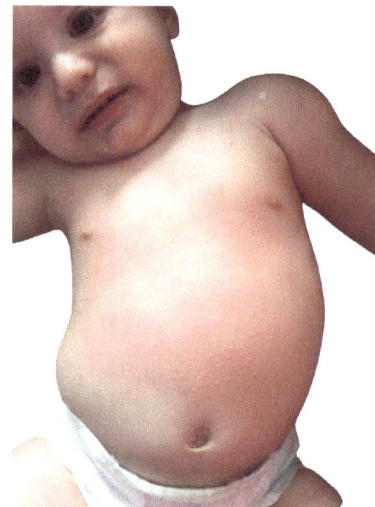

70

SEPSIS[13]

- "Life threatening organ dysfunction caused by a dysregulated host response to an infection."
    - Cytokine release
    - Malperfusion
    - Massive loss of vascular tone
        - Septic shock
        - Increased capillary permeability
- Leading cause of mortality in infection

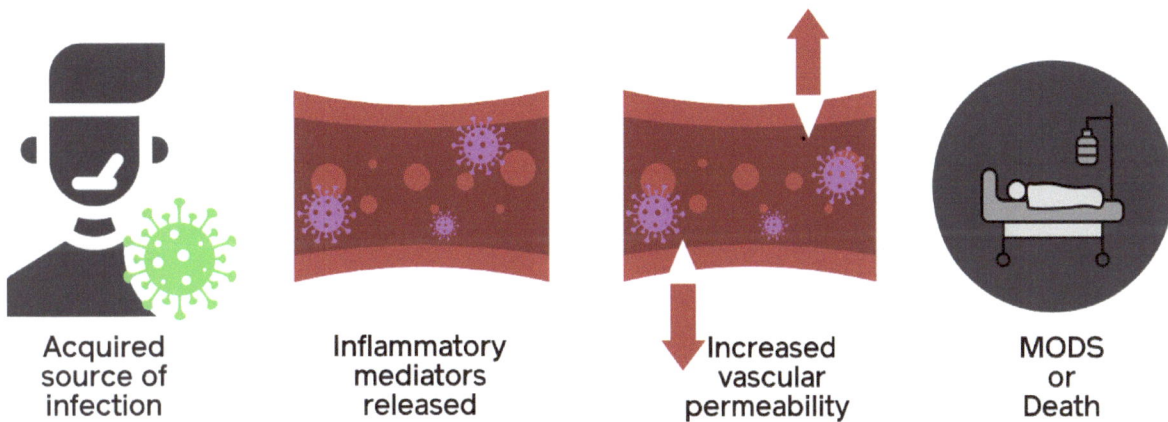

Acquired source of infection

Inflammatory mediators released

Increased vascular permeability

MODS or Death

Increased capillary permeability and vasodilation causes distributive shock

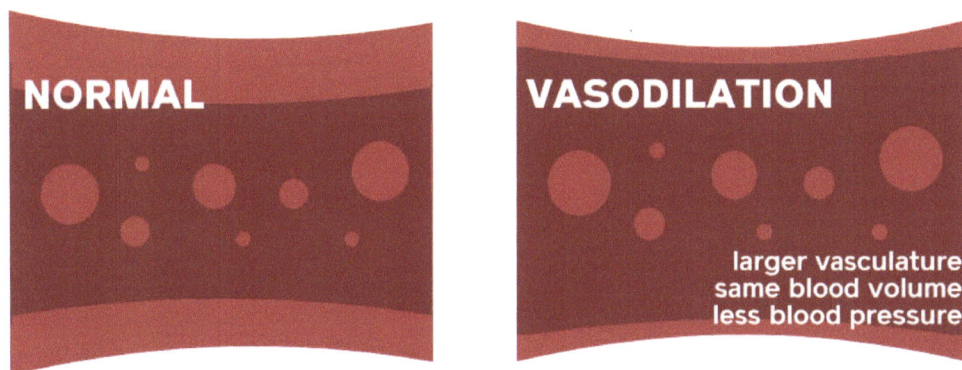

NORMAL

VASODILATION

larger vasculature
same blood volume
less blood pressure

Sepsis Related Organ Failure Assessment Tool (qSOFA)[2,13]

- GCS <13
- SBP <100 mmHg
- Respirations >22

Treatment: "Sepsis Bundle"[2,13]

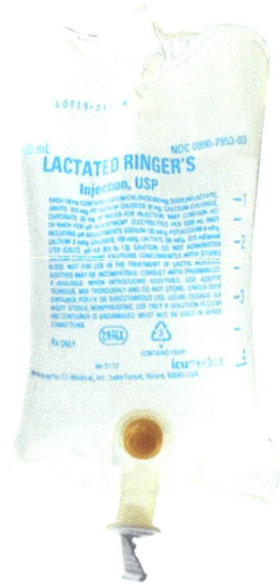

30mL/kg
Lactated Ringers Preferred

Early Pressors
Levophed, Epi, Vasopressin, Phenelephrine

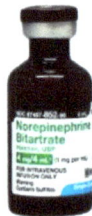

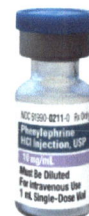

Antibiotics
Broad Spectrum Preferred

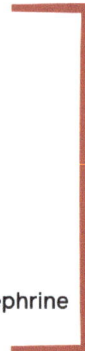

MAP GOAL
>65mmHg

Vasopressors in Septic Shock[15]

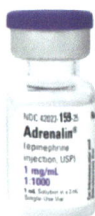

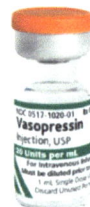

1	2	3	4
Norepinephrine	**Epinephrine**	**Vasopressin**	**Phenylephrine**
Alpha effect, some beta	Alpha and beta effects	Vasoconstriction, water retention	Pure alpha, vasoconstriction

RENAL PATHOLOGY

Acute Renal Failure[6]
- **Rise in serum creatinine or decline in urine output within hours to days**
- **Labs:**
  - **Creatinine increase of >0.3 mg/dL or 1.5x baseline**
  - **Increased BUN**
  - **Hyperkalemia**
- **Edema**

Types of ARF[6]
- **Prerenal: pathology BEFORE the kidney**
  - **Hypoperfusion of kidneys**
- **Intrarenal: pathology WITHIN the kidney**
  - **Intrinsic kidney disease**
  - **Rhabdomyolysis**
  - **Toxicity (ibuprofen overuse, etc.)**
- **Postrenal: pathology AFTER the kidney**
  - **Obstruction**

Rhabdomyolysis
- **Excessive muscle breakdown, causing myoglobinemia**
  - **Crush injuries**
  - **Extended down time post fall**
  - **Exertional**
- **Presents with Coke-colored urine, extreme muscle pain, edema**
- **Elevated CK**
  - **Mild: 1,000-5,000 u/L**
  - **Moderate: 5,000-15,000 u/L**
  - **Severe: >15,000 u/L**

Rhabdomyolysis Treatment
- **Fluid administration**
  - **LR**
  - **Titrate fluids to maintain 100mL/hour urine output**
- **Dialysis in severe cases**
- **Protect patient from nephrotoxins**

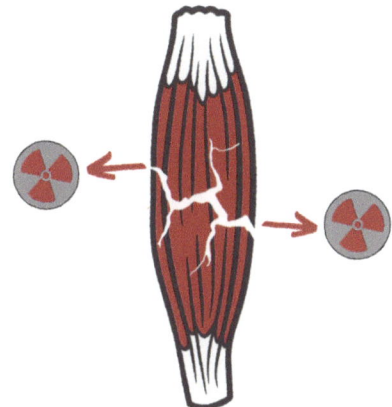

ABDOMINAL PATHOLOGY

GI Bleeding[12,14]
- **Upper (UGIB)**
  - **Presents with: hematemesis, melena**
  - **Causes: Esophageal varices, excessive vomiting, peptic ulcer disease, Mallory-Wiess tear**
- **Lower (LGIB)**
  - **Presents with: hematochezia**
  - **Causes: colitis, Crohn's, diverticulitis, internal hemorrhoids**

Treatment of GI Bleeding[11,12,14]
- **Blood transfusion**
- **Antibiotics**
- **Proton Pump Inhibitors**
- **TXA**
- **Octreotide**

Esophageal Varices[14]
- **Results from late stages of portal hypertension**
- **Life threatening hemorrhage requires tamponade tube: Minnesota or Blakemore**

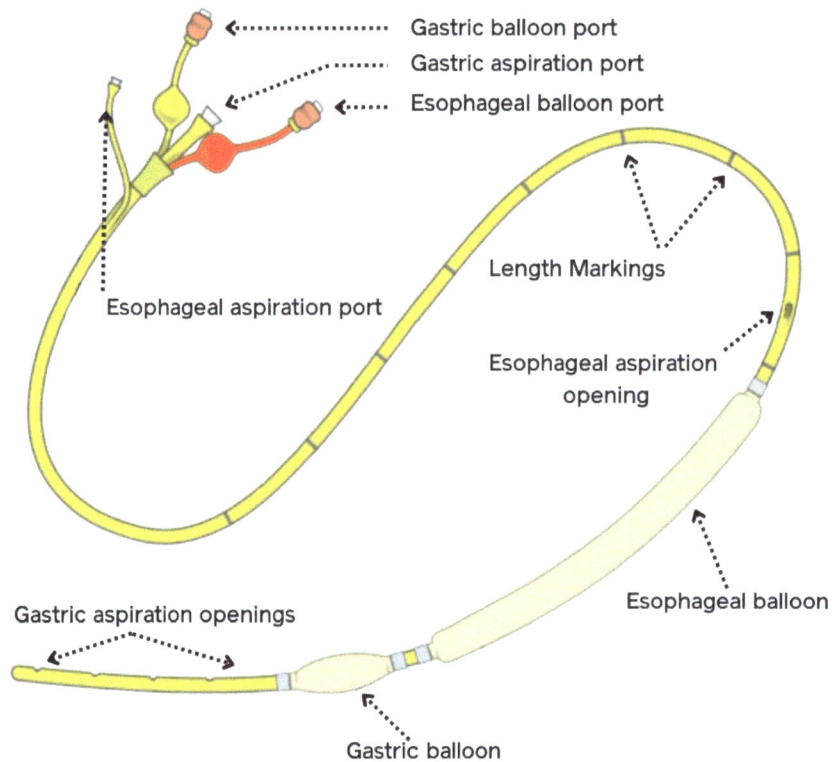

Pancreatitis[17]

- **Presents with: epigastric pain, n/v, inflammatory ileus, elevated amylase (3x baseline) and lipase**
- **Inflammatory**
    - **Caused by: gallstones, chronic alcohol abuse, ERCP complications**
- **Necrotizing**
    - **Dysregulated caustic secretions**
    - **MODS, SIRS**

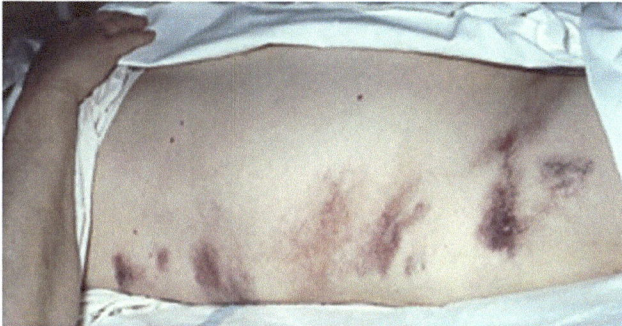

Hendrik A. van Dijk. Open Access license: Wikimedia commons

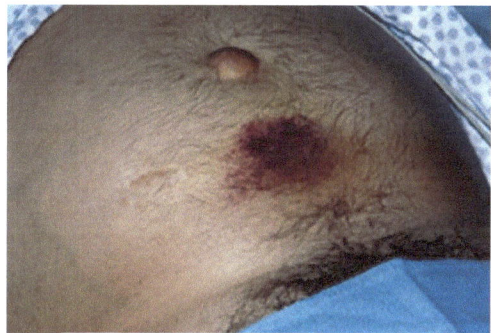

Images: Herbert L. Fred, MD and

Grey Turner Sign

Disorders of the Spleen[1,12]

- **Presents with Kehr's sign: referred pain to left shoulder**
- **Causes: splenomegaly, atrial fibrillation**

Bowel Problems[12]

- **Ileus**
- **Diverticulitis**
    - **LUQ pain**
    - **Usually constant and present for days**
- **Colitis: bloody diarrhea, colicky abdominal pain**
- **Crohn's Disease**
    - **Variable symptoms for years**
    - **Fatigue**
    - **Prolonged diarrhea with weight loss**

Appendicitis[1,12]

- **Periumbilical pain that radiates to RUQ**
- **Rebound tenderness**
- **McBurney's Point**
- **Surgery vs. antibiotics**

Mesenteric Ischemia[10]
- 80% mortality
- Vague signs and symptoms
- Subtle and vague CT findings

Abdominal Compartment Syndrome[6]
- Primarily affects critical ICU patients
- Tensely distended abdomen
- Abdomen pushes on mediastinum compressing heart
- Causes increased PIP and MAP
- Compresses renal vasculature
- Decompression: huge risk v. benefit analysis

questions:

1. The patient is a 35-year-old female with no past medical or psychiatric history. Her husband called 911 after she pulled a hose into the house and began to spray the walls screaming that the house was on fire. He is adamant that she is healthy but stated that she has been very tired for the past two weeks which is abnormal. Her vital signs are Pulse 130, RR 28, BP 86/42, SpO2 99%, Temp 103.1. You suspect:

    a. Sepsis
    b. Urinary tract infection
    c. Myxedema coma
    d. Thyroid Storm

2. The patient is a 45-year-old female who is 3 weeks status post-surgery to remove a glioblastoma. She presents with tachypnea, tachycardia, and she is lying in a bed that is soaked with urine. The most likely etiology is:

    a. Thyroid Storm
    b. HHNK
    c. Diabetes Insipidus
    d. Osmotic hypertension

Chapter 6 CITATIONS:

1. AAOS. (2022). Nancy Caroline's Emergency Care in the Streets. 9th Ed.
2. Bakker J. Lactate is THE target for early resuscitation in sepsis. Rev Bras Ter Intensiva. 2017 Apr-Jun;29(2):124-127. doi: 10.5935/0103-507X.20170021. PMID: 28977252; PMCID: PMC5496745.
3. Balcı AK, Koksal O, Kose A, Armagan E, Ozdemir F, Inal T, Oner N. General characteristics of patients with electrolyte imbalance admitted to emergency department. World J Emerg Med. 2013;4(2):113-6. doi: 10.5847/wjem.j.issn.1920-8642.2013.02.005. PMID: 25215103; PMCID: PMC4129840.
4. Josh Farkas. (2021). Hyperkalemia. IBCC. Available: https://emcrit.org/ibcc/hyperkalemia/
5. Farkas, Josh. (2021). Thyroid Storm. IBCC. Available from: https://emcrit.org/ibcc/tstorm/#top
6. Fatehi, Pedram, Hsu, Chi-yuan. (2022). Evaluation of Acute Kidney Injury Among Hospitalized Adult Patients. Up-to-Date.
7. Gestring, Mark. (2022). Abdominal Compartment Syndrome in Adults. Up-to-Date.
8. Hirsch, Irl. Emmett, Michael. (2022). Diabetic Ketoacidosis and Hyperosmolar Hyperglycemic State in Adults: Treatment. Up-to-Date.
9. Hui C, Khan M, Radbel JM. Diabetes Insipidus. [Updated 2022 Aug 12]. In: StatPearls [Internet]. Treasure Island (FL): StatPearls Publishing; 2022 Jan-. Available from: https://www.ncbi.nlm.nih.gov/books/NBK470458/
10. Kärkkäinen JM. Acute Mesenteric Ischemia: A Challenge for the Acute Care Surgeon. Scand J Surg. 2021 Jun;110(2):150-158. doi: 10.1177/14574969211007590. Epub 2021 Apr 19. PMID: 33866891; PMCID: PMC8258713.
11. Noveloso B, Bastiampillai B, Perni N, Waterman A. Antibiotic Prophylaxis in Patients with Cirrhosis and Upper Gastrointestinal Bleeding. Am Fam Physician. 2017 May 1;95(9):582. PMID: 28671382.
12. Penner, R. and Fishman, M. (2022). Causes of Abdominal Pain in Adults. Up-to-Date
13. Purcarea A, Sovaila S. Sepsis, a 2020 review for the internist. Rom J Intern Med. 2020 Sep 1;58(3):129-137. doi: 10.2478/rjim-2020-0012. PMID: 32396142.
14. Saltzman, John. (2022). Approach to acute upper gastrointestinal bleeding in adults. Up-to-Date.
15. Shi R, Hamzaoui O, De Vita N, Monnet X, Teboul JL. Vasopressors in septic shock: which, when, and how much? Ann Transl Med. 2020 Jun;8(12):794. doi: 10.21037/atm.2020.04.24. PMID: 32647719; PMCID: PMC7333107.
16. Shrimanker I, Bhattarai S. Electrolytes. [Updated 2022 Jul 25]. In: StatPearls [Internet]. Treasure Island (FL): StatPearls Publishing; 2022 Jan-. Available from: https://www.ncbi.nlm.nih.gov/books/NBK541123/
17. Vege, Santhi. (2022). Clinical Manifestations and Diagnosis of Acute Pancreatitis. Up-to-Date.
18. PMID 22909382, 22028373, 2934126
19. Mejia (Ed.). (2022, April 8). Critical Care Transport (3rd ed.). Jones and Bartlett Learning

CHAPTER 7: TOXICOLOGY

Toxicosis Effects:
- Speeds up or slows down metabolism
- Increases or decreases pH
- Causes alterations in mental status

THE INITIAL PATIENT CARE PRIORITY IN ALL TOXIDROMES IS SUPPORTIVE CARE.

Poison Control Center: 1-800-222-1222
- Poison control should be contacted for every toxic exposure/overdose patient
  - Patient demographics and history
  - Current status
  - Offending agent
  - Time of exposure
  - Route of exposure
  - Amount ingested

ACETAMINOPHEN TOXICITY (TYLENOL)

STAGE 1:
Malaise, RUQ pain (0-24hrs)

STAGE 2:
Elevated liver labs (18-72hrs)

STAGE 3:
Maximal Liver Injury (72-96hrs)

STAGE 4:
Recovery (4-21 days)

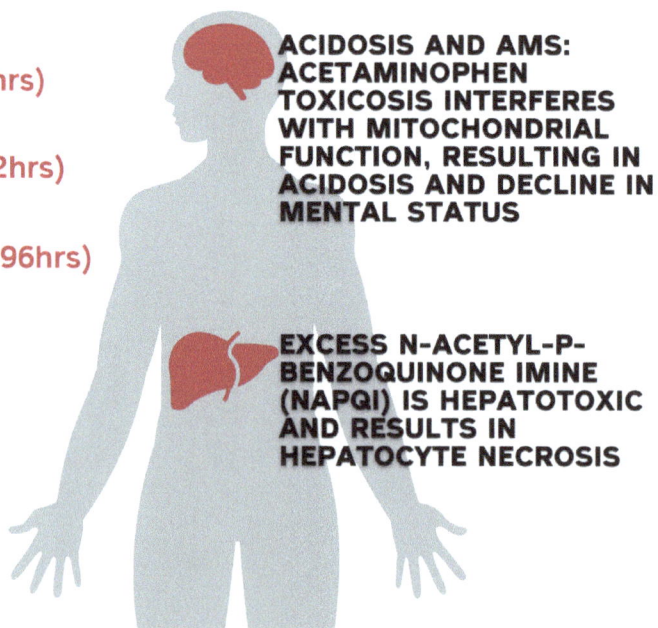

ACIDOSIS AND AMS: ACETAMINOPHEN TOXICOSIS INTERFERES WITH MITOCHONDRIAL FUNCTION, RESULTING IN ACIDOSIS AND DECLINE IN MENTAL STATUS

EXCESS N-ACETYL-P-BENZOQUINONE IMINE (NAPQI) IS HEPATOTOXIC AND RESULTS IN HEPATOCYTE NECROSIS

- N-Acetylcysteine[1, 2, 3]
  Binds with the toxic metabolites of acetaminophen
- Should be given within 8-10 hours of ingestion for maximal effectiveness
  - Dose based on serum acetaminophen levels, time from ingestion, and patient weight

Outcomes in Acetaminophen Toxicity[1,2,3]
- 7.2% of overdoses cause acute liver failure
  - 10% of these cases advance to severe liver failure
  - Most patients recover with n-acetylcysteine (NAC)
  - Death is rare with early NAC administration
  - Indications for liver transplant:
  - Arterial pH >7.3
  - INR >6.5
  - Crt >3.4
  - High grade encephalopathy

ACETYLSALICYLIC ACID TOXICITY (ASPIRIN)[4]

- There is no antidote
- Management is focused on preventing further absorption and increasing elimination
- First acid-base imbalance: respiratory alkalosis
  - Late: metabolic acidosis
- Symptoms
  - Early: burning in mouth, malaise, N/V, dizziness, tinnitus
  - Moderate: tachypnea, hyperpyrexia, sweating, dehydration, ataxia, restlessness
  - Severe: hallucinations, stupor, cerebral edema, seizures, renal failure, cardiovascular collapse
- Treatment
  - ICU: sodium bicarbonate
  - Hemodialysis

BETA BLOCKER AND CALCIUM CHANNEL BLOCKER TOXICITY

Beta Blocker Toxicity[5]
- Isolated beta blocker toxicity is uncommon
  - Isolated overdose is usually intentional
- Hallmark symptoms are cardiovascular
- Most common: bradycardia and hypotension*
- Check blood glucose, may cause hypoglycemia

Calcium Channel Blocker Toxicity[6]
- Directly inhibits voltage in myocardial calcium channels
- CCB's cause vasodilation
  - Distributive shock
- Onset may be delayed by hours
- May impair insulin release and cause hyperglycemia

Treatment of Beta Blocker and Calcium Channel Blocker Overdose[6]
- Pharmacotherapy is aimed at improving bradycardia and myocardial contractility
- High-dose insulin for positive inotropy
- Catecholamines are complementary (but effective) therapy
- High-dose glucagon may be of some benefit

BENZODIAZEPINE TOXICITY[12]
- Alters the use of GABA
- Isolated benzo overdose is rare
- Hallmark clinical findings of isolated benzo OD:
  - CNS depression
  - Normal or near-normal VS
  - AMS with slurred speech and ataxia but arousable
- Children have signs and symptoms within 4 hours of ingestion
- Ataxia is the most common sign of a benzodiazepine overdose in peds
- Treat with supportive care

Flumazenil (Romazicon) for Benzodiazepine Overdose[12]
- Competitive antagonist for benzodiazepines
- Very risky to administer
- May cause precipitous withdrawal
- Risks usually outweigh the benefits

OPIATE TOXICITY[13]
- Heroin epidemic
- Synthetic opioids: 70% increase in mortality

Buprenorphine[13]
- Recovery medication
- Unlikely to cause respiratory depression
- Peds: may see respiratory depression and delayed onset

Loperamide[13]
- Binds to opiate receptors in the GI tract
- High doses produce a "high"
- Causes QT prolongation

Gabapentin[13]
- Chronic opiate use and gabapentin often go hand-in-hand
- 15% of opiate users report using gabapentin to get high

Kratom[13]
- Opiate-like in high doses
- May cause seizures
- Responds to naloxone and benzodiazepines

STIMULANTS: COCAINE, METHAMPHETAMINE[15]
- Clinical findings: CV complications, psychosis, delirium
- Cocaine users more likely to present to ED with trauma
- Methamphetamine was more likely to present with AMS
- Avg HR: 106
- Avg BP: 142/90
- BNP higher with meth users

TOXIC ALCOHOL POISONING[7]
- HALLMARK SIGN IS WIDE GAP METABOLIC ACIDOSIS
- High serum osmolality
- Hepatic toxic: liver metabolizes toxic alcohols
- Renal toxic: kidney excretes them
- Dialysis is highly effective at toxic alcohol elimination

Methanol[7]
- Visual disturbances
- Abdominal pain, pancreatitis

Ethylene Glycol[7]
- Identification is often delayed
- Calcium oxalate crystals found in brain, heart, lung tissue on autopsy

- **Kussmaul's breathing is seen at all stages**
- **Cerebral edema**

Isopropanol (Rubbing Alcohol)[7]
- Has direct effects on organ tissue
- Toxic to gastric tissue

Treatment of Toxic Alcohols[7]
- Administration of ethanol alcohol or Fomepizole
  - Both Inhibit alcohol dehydrogenase (ADH)
- Fomepizole has greater affinity for ADH than ETOH
- Fomepizole does not cause slowing of metabolism

ETHANOL ALCOHOL[9]
- Beer Potomania: Dilutional hyponatremia from drinking too much beer
- Alcoholic Ketoacidosis[10]
  - Lethargy
  - Tachycardia
  - Dehydration
  - Abdominal pain
  - Agitation, lethargy
  - Ketone odor
  - Tachypnea

TRICYCLIC ANTIDEPRESSANT (TCA) TOXICITY[11]

TCA Toxic Effects:
- Inhibits norepinephrine reuptake
- Direct alpha block
- Membrane stabilizing effect on myocardium (too much)
- Anticholinergic reaction

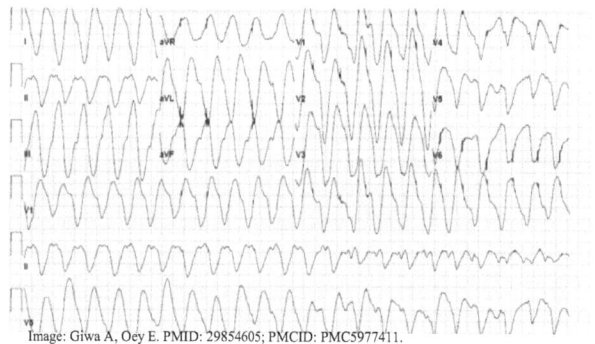

Image: Giwa A, Oey E. PMID: 29854605; PMCID: PMC5977411.

Clinical Features of TCA Overdose[11]
- Wide QRS
- Hyperthermia with impaired sweating
- Hypotension
- Coma in 17%

TCA overdose: Treatment[11]
- Sodium bicarbonate: cardiac stabilization
- Norepinephrine
- ECMO
- Do not give activated charcoal (ineffective)

CARDIAC GLYCOSIDES: DIGITALIS[14]
- **GI distress is usually the first symptom**
- **Often vague symptoms**
- **May see green or yellow halos around objects**
- **Treated with Digibind (digoxin immune fab)**
- **Characteristic EKG changes:**
  - **Slowing heart rate**
  - **ST depression described as "ice cream scoop" in appearance**

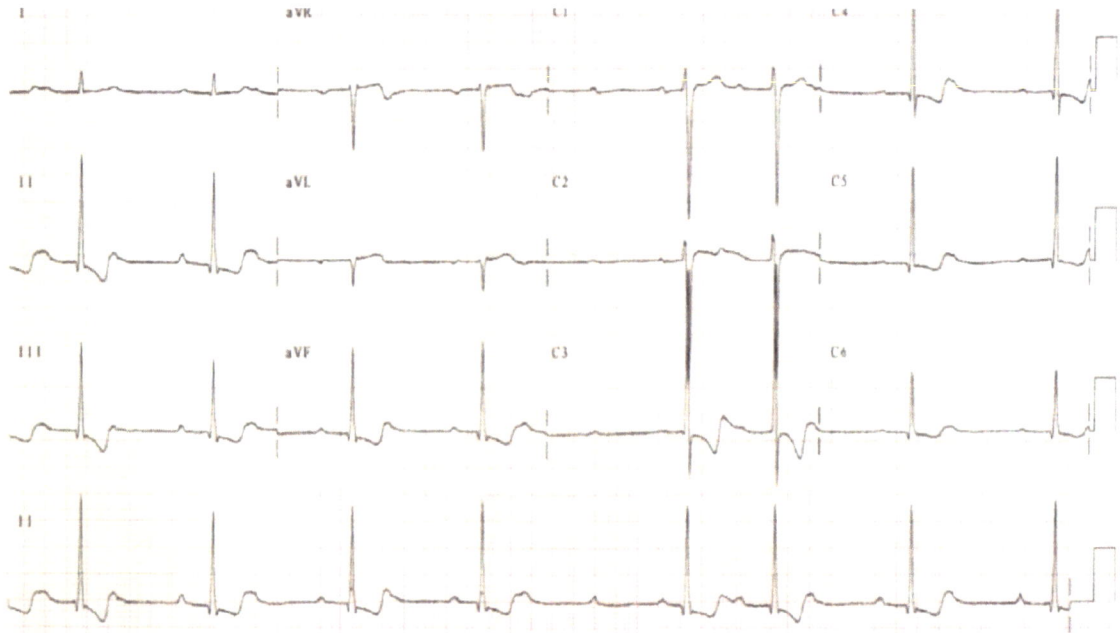

EKG Image: Heather Wetherall. (2015). Digoxin and the heart. Br. J. Cardiology, 22: 96-7.

questions:

1. **Your patient has a wide-gap metabolic acidosis with AMS of unknown etiology. You suspect:**

   a. **Fomepizole poisoning**
   b. **TCA overdose**
   c. **Digitalis poisoning**
   d. **Ethylene glycol toxicity**

2. **The first acid/base derangement noted in Aspirin poisoning is:**

   a. **Metabolic acidosis**
   b. **Metabolic alkalosis**
   c. **Respiratory acidosis**
   d. **Respiratory alkalosis**

Chapter 7 CITATIONS:

1. PMID 34053705
2. PMID 35440504
3. PMID 22998987
4. Dargan PI, Wallace CI, Jones AL. An evidence based flowchart to guide the management of acute salicylate (aspirin) overdose. Emerg Med J. 2002 May;19(3):206-9. doi: 10.1136/emj.19.3.206. PMID: 11971828; PMCID: PMC1725844.
5. Lauterbach M. Clinical toxicology of beta-blocker overdose in adults. Basic Clin Pharmacol Toxicol. 2019 Aug;125(2):178-186. doi: 10.1111/bcpt.13231. Epub 2019 Apr 15. PMID: 30916882.
6. Graudins A, Lee HM, Druda D. Calcium channel antagonist and beta-blocker overdose: antidotes and adjunct therapies. Br J Clin Pharmacol. 2016 Mar;81(3):453-61. doi: 10.1111/bcp.12763. Epub 2015 Oct 30. PMID: 26344579; PMCID: PMC4767195.
7. Kraut JA, Kurtz I. Toxic alcohol ingestions: clinical features, diagnosis, and management. Clin
8. J Am Soc Nephrol. 2008 Jan;3(1):208-25. doi: 10.2215/CJN.03220807. Epub 2007 Nov 28. PMID: 18045860.
9. Joshi R, Chou SY. Beer Potomania: A View on the Dynamic Process of Developing Hyponatremia. Cureus. 2018 Jul 22;10(7):e3024. doi: 10.7759/cureus.3024. PMID: 30254813; PMCID: PMC6150768
10. Howard RD, Bokhari SRA. Alcoholic Ketoacidosis. 2022 May 8. In: StatPearls [Internet]. Treasure Island (FL): StatPearls Publishing; 2022 Jan–. PMID: 28613672.
11. Kerr GW, McGuffie AC, Wilkie S. Tricyclic antidepressant overdose: a review. Emerg Med J. 2001 Jul;18(4):236-41. doi: 10.1136/emj.18.4.236. PMID: 11435353; PMCID: PMC1725608
12. Kang M, Galuska MA, Ghassemzadeh S. Benzodiazepine Toxicity. [Updated 2022 Jun 27]. In: StatPearls [Internet]. Treasure Island (FL): StatPearls Publishing; 2022 Jan- . Available from: https://www.ncbi.nlm.nih.gov/books/NBK482238/
13. Toce MS, Chai PR, Burns MM, Boyer EW. Pharmacologic Treatment of Opioid Use Disorder: a Review of Pharmacotherapy, Adjuncts, and Toxicity. J Med Toxicol. 2018 Dec;14(4):306-322. doi: 10.1007/s13181-018-0685-1. Epub 2018 Oct 30. PMID: 30377951; PMCID: PMC6242798.
14. Cummings ED, Swoboda HD. Digoxin Toxicity. [Updated 2022 Jul 4]. In: StatPearls [Internet]. Treasure Island (FL): StatPearls Publishing; 2022 Jan-. Available from: https://www.ncbi.nlm.nih.gov/books/NBK470568/
15. Richards, J., Tabish, N. (2017). Cocaine vs methamphetamine users in the ED: How do they differ? J. Alcohol and Drug Dependence, 5(3).

CHAPTER 8: FLIGHT PHYSIOLOGY

Dalton's Law[1]

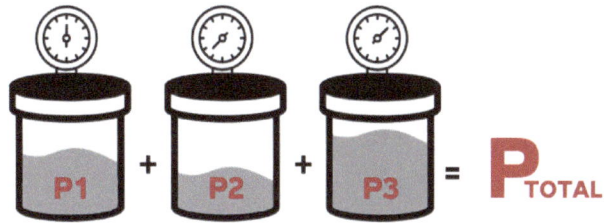

THE TOTAL PRESSURE OF A MIXTURE OF GASES EQUALS THE PARTIAL PRESSURE EXERTED BY EACH GAS

Boyle's Law[1,2]
- For a given temperature the volume is inversely proportional to the pressure
- Volume decreases as pressure increases
- Volume increases as pressure decreases (altitude)

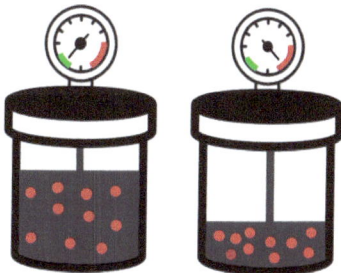

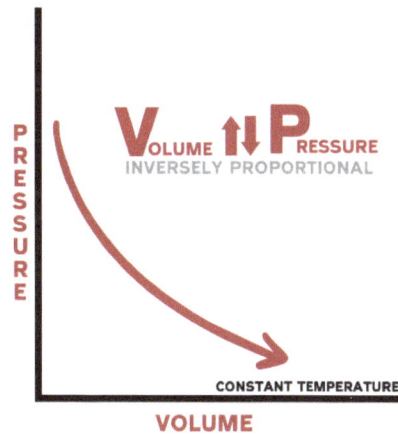

Effects of Boyle's Law (Trapped Gas)[4]
- **Gastrointestinal distress**
- **Ear pain: expanding pressure in middle ear**
- **Sinus pain: trapped gases during flight**
- **Barodontalgia**
- **ETT cuff pressure**

Charles's Law[1]
- **For a given pressure, the volume is proportional to the temperature**
- **Gas expands when it is heated**

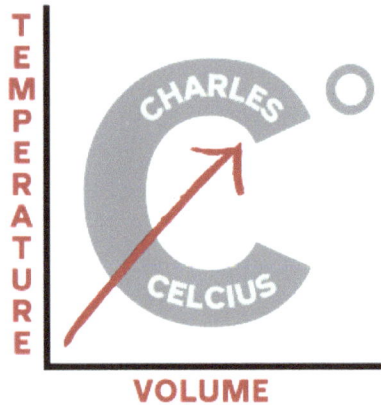

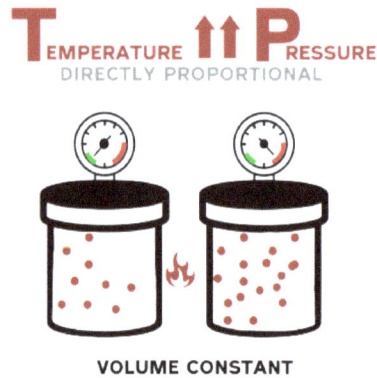

Gay-Lussac's Law[2]
- **The pressure of a fixed mass of gas at a constant volume is directly proportional to its absolute temperature**
- **Application: for every 1000ft of altitude, the temperature decreases $1^{\circ}C$ (or 330 ft for $1^{\circ}F$)**

Henry's Law
- **The amount of given gas dissolved in a liquid is directly proportional to the partial pressure of the gas in contact with the liquid**
- **Decompression Sickness[4]**
  - **Rapid ascent: body does not have time to acclimate**
  - **Nitrogen tends to form bubbles in the tissues and blood**
  - **Type I DCS: "The Bends"**
  - **Type II DCS: "The Chokes"**

HYPOXIA: TYPES AND STAGES[3]

Hypoxic Hypoxia
- **Most common cause in flight (aka: altitude hypoxia)**
- **Inadequate ambient oxygen**

Hypemic Hypoxia
- **Reduced capacity of the blood to carry oxygen**
  - **Carbon monoxide reduces the hemoglobin's ability to carry O_2**

Stagnant Hypoxia
- **Inadequate blood flow causes insufficient tissue oxygenation**
- **Shock states leading to sluggish blood flow**

Histotoxic Hypoxia
- The cell is unable to use oxygen
- Cyanide poisoning

Stages of Hypoxia[4]
- Indifferent (90-98%)
- Compensatory (80-89%)
- Disturbance (70-79%)
- Critical (60-69%)

STRESSORS OF AIR TRANSPORT

Self-Imposed Stressors[3]
- Medications
- Supplements
- Energy Drinks
- Tobacco, nicotine
- Alcohol

Effects of Nicotine[7]
- Experiences effects of hypoxia at lower altitudes
- Increased CO level
- Nicotine affects vision
    - Reduced night vision
    - 40% reduction in night vision at 5,000' MSL

Alcohol Consumption
- 14 CFR 91.17
- No person may act as a crew member of a civil aircraft
    - Within 8 hours after consumption of any alcoholic beverage
    - While under the influence of alcohol

Fatigue[3]
- Circadian effects
- Physical fatigue
- Recommendations:
    - Breaks of 15 min every 2 hours
    - Schedule 24 hours of uninterrupted rest after night shifts
    - Schedule off days in periods of at least three days
    - Exercise, diet, no smoking

Vibration[6]
- Rotor wing transport causes whole-body vibration
  - Motion sickness
  - Hyperventilation
  - Headache
  - Decreased visual acuity
- May cause acceleration of spine disorders
- Causes localized leg, buttocks, and back pain with numbness and muscle spasms

Flicker Vertigo[5]
- Confuses the vestibular system
- May result in spatial disorientation leading to inaccurate perceptions of altitude, and speed

Pressurized vs. Unpressurized Cabins

CFR 91.211: Supplemental oxygen must be worn by pilot:
- At >12,500 MSL for >30 min
- At >14,000 MSL during the entire time at altitude for "required minimum flight crew"
- >15,000 MSL: oxygen must be worn by everyone on board or cabin must be pressurized

Physiologic Zones

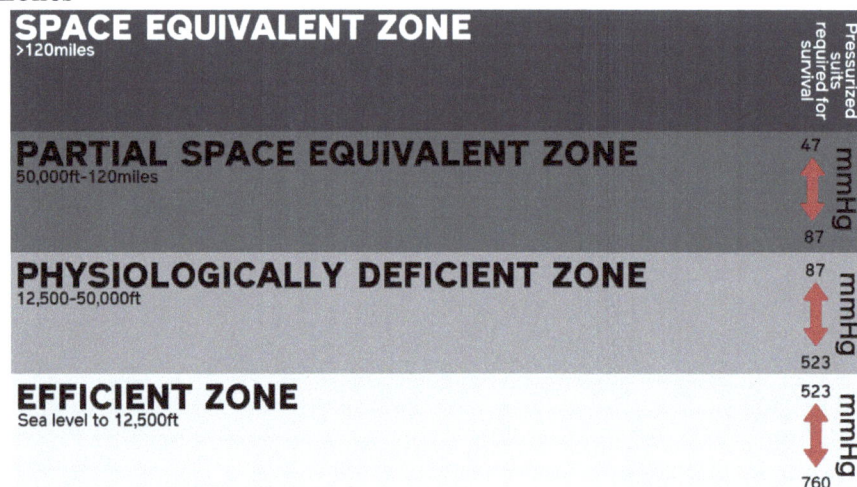

Time of Useful Consciousness (TUC)[3]
- The time between the interruption of oxygen and the time a pilot is unable to perform flying duties effectively
  - Slow loss of pressure at 30,000' altitude: 90 seconds
  - Rapid depressurization at 30,000' altitude: 45 seconds

QUESTIONS:

1. Which of the following stressors will make the aircrew member particularly susceptible to flicker vertigo?

    a. Consumption of an energy drink before the flight
    b. Consumption of a mixed drink 15 hours prior
    c. Consumption of nicotine products
    d. Psychosocial stress

2. An aircraft flying at 20,000 MSL has experienced a depressurization of the cabin. The co-pilot tells the PIC who does not immediately respond to verbal commands that the aircraft should descend. The PIC nods in affirmation but speaks incoherently and is unable to maintain controls due to loss of dexterity. The PIC is exhibiting which stage of hypoxia?

    a. Indifferent
    b. Compensatory
    c. Disturbance
    d. Critical

Chapter 8 citations:

1. Tarver, W., Volner, K., & Cooper, J. (2022, October 24). Aerospace Pressure Effects. National Library of Medicine. https://www.ncbi.nlm.nih.gov/books/NBK470190/
2. Yartsev, A. (n.d.). Common respiratory equations. Deranged Physiology. https://derangedphysiology.com/main/cicm-primary-exam/required-reading/respiratory-system/Chapter+133/common-respiratory-equations
3. Boshers, L. (2015, July 21). Beware of Hypoxia. faa.gov. https://www.faa.gov/pilots/training/airman_education/topics_of_interest/hypoxia
4. Aeromedical Training for Flight Personnel. (2019, January 22). armypubs.army.mil. https://armypubs.army.mil/epubs/DR_pubs/DR_a/pdf/web/ARN14652_TC%203-04x93%20C1%20INC%20FINAL%20WEB.pdf
5. CFR 91.211
6. Awareness of Causes and Symptoms of Flicker Vertigo Can Limit Ill Effects. (2004). Flight Safety Foundation, 51(5). https://flightsafety.org/hf/hf_mar-apr04.pdf

CHAPTER 9: FLIGHT AND SURFACE OPERATIONS

CAMTS
- Accrediting body for flight and ground transport programs
- Performs audits and site surveys
- CAMTS standards:
  - ¼" space between skin and flight suit
  - 4 flight ready pilots for 1 aircraft operating 24/7
  - Pilots must have 2000 hours, 1000 as PIC, 100 at night

FAR Part 135: "Air Taxi"
- Applies to all flights conducted for compensation
- PIC is ultimate authority
- Maximum 14-hour day for pilots
  - Max 8 hours flight time in one day
- 8 hours "bottle to throttle"
- Passengers must be provided safety briefing

Local Area vs. Cross Country[8]
- "Local flying area" must be well defined by geographic or manmade features as defined by the certificate holder
- Cross country flights are those outside of the local area

14 CFR 91.107: Safety Belts
- No pilot may move the aircraft unless each person has been notified to fasten his or her safety belt and, if installed, his or her shoulder harness
- Children under 2: may be held by an adult who is occupying an approved seat or berth

Child Restraint Systems[9]
- (Pt weight in pounds) x speed = force needed to restrain
- 25 lbs x 35 mph = 875 lbs of restraint
- National Association of State EMS Officials has an approved list of available restraint devices
- Ensure that child's weight and height are both in the specified range for the device

Surface Transport Safety Belts[10]
- Ambulance personnel must be seat belted when the ambulance is in motion unless emergent patient condition precludes it
- Side facing bench seats are not recommended
- If the ambulance has side facing bench seats, seat belt mountings must be situated at the pelvic level in order to restrain personnel/passengers

Dispatching Flight Requests
- The dispatch information should contain NO information about the type of incident, patient, or acuity
- Example: "Scene request for Sussex County. Coordinates: 39.52.09/74.35.02. Estimated weight: 120 kg. Ground contact is on S-Fire-2."

Mission Safety Decisions
- "Three to go, one to say no"
- Pushing weather is one of the chief causes of accidents
- Illusion of groupthink
- "Put your manager hat on"

Risk Assessment Tools[5]
- We incorporate our desires and biases in making decisions that involve some degree of risk
- PAVE Checklist:
  Pilot
  Aircraft
  enVironment
  External pressures

Flight Following & Operational Control[8]
- Satellite tracking systems strongly recommended
- Rotor: 15-minute position checks*
- Surface: Time must not exceed 45 minutes while on ground without communication*
  - *Unless continuous GPS tracking is utilized

Post-Accident Incident Plan (PAIP)[8]
- Transport-tracking protocol requires PAIP so that appropriate search and rescue efforts may be initiated if:
  - The transport vehicle is overdue
  - Radio communications cannot be established
  - Location cannot be verified

Walk Arounds
- "FOD": Foreign Object Debris
- FAA AC 150/5120-24: any object, live or not, located in an inappropriate location in the airport environment that has the capacity to injure airport or airport carrier personnel and damage aircraft

VFR and IFR

- **VFR: maintain aircraft control by visual cues**
- **14 CFR 91.155: VFR weather minimums**
  - **Day: 1 mile visibility, 500 feet**
  - **Night: 3 miles visibility, 500 feet**

Inadvertent Instrument Meteorologic Conditions (IIMC)[2]

- **Pilot unprepared by the loss of visual reference**
- **Many accidents can be traced back to the pilot's inability to regain control in IIMC**
- **Aircrew member may be charged with watching controls**

Ground Transport Risk Management[6]

- **Ground transport can be just as risky as flight and should be using risk assessment tools**

Crew Resource Management[1]

- **"A team member's awareness of how their action or inaction affects the safe operation of the flight."**
- **"A superior pilot uses his or her superior judgement to avoid situations requiring his or her superior skill."**
- **Orville Wright: "What is needed is better judgement rather than better skill."**
- **"SEE IT. SAY IT. FIX IT."**

CRM Tenants

- **Leveling of hierarchies when safety concerns arise**
- **Agreement on near-term objectives**
- **Consideration of all available options**
- **Workload management/delegation**
- **Monitor and evaluate results**

Critical Phases of Flight

- **Takeoff and landing**
- **Refueling**
- **Taxi**
- **Traveling through busy/controlled airspace**

FAR 121.542/135.100 – Sterile Cockpit

- **No crew member may engage (and the PIC may not permit), any activity during a critical phase of flight that could interfere with proper conduct of flight duties**
- **No non-essential conversations or functions (e.g., eating meals)**
- **Any conversation is required to be related to the safe operation of the aircraft**

Laser Strikes[11]

- **2021: 9,723 laser strikes**
- **High powered lasers can incapacitate pilots**
- **Penalties of up to $11,000 per violation**

- FAA has a laser incident reporting form

LANDING ZONE: MINIMUM REQUREMENTS
- Secured, illuminated
- Free of overhead and ground obstructions
- Free of debris
- As level as possible

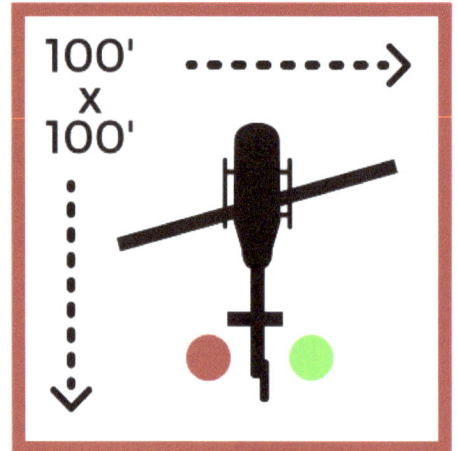

HELICOPTER APPROACH AND EMERGENCY PROCEDURES
- Never approach from the rear
- Do not travel uphill from aircraft
- If emergency egress, meet at 12 o'clock position

Categories of In-Flight Emergencies
- Land immediately
- Land as soon as possible
- Land as soon as practicable

Emergency Shut Down Procedures
Order of shut down in the event of an emergency:
- Throttle
- Fuel
- Battery
- Brake (Rotor)

Memory helper for this order:
"This Freakin' B*tch Broke!"

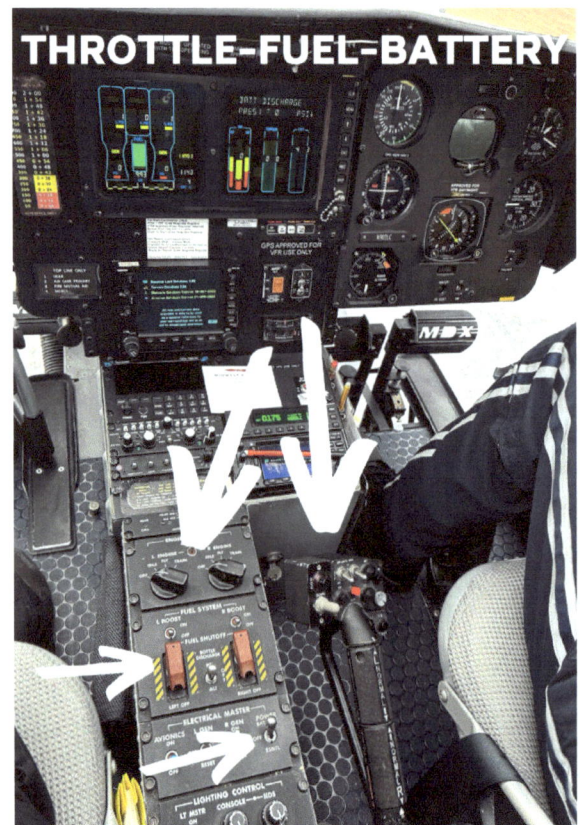

Night Vision Goggles[4]
- Enhance operational safety and situation awareness
- Increase ability to see obstructions
- Increased helmet weight
- Depth and peripheral vision deficits

CAMTS: Survival Standards[10]
- The transport vehicle must be equipped with survival gear appropriate to coverage area and the number of occupants.
- Survival gear must have expiration dates and be checked at appropriate intervals

Emergency Locator Transmitter (ELT):
- 406 MHz
- 121.5 MHz
- Manual activation
- 4 g-force activation

RADIO SYSTEMS
- Ultra-High Frequency: Lower range but penetrate barriers well
- Very High Frequency: Longer range
- Trunked systems (700, 800 mHz)

SURFACE OPERATIONS

Ambulance Standards[14]
- Must meet KKK 1822 standards or state licensure requirements in place at the time the vehicle was built:
  - Adequate interior lighting
  - Capability of shielding cab from light
  - Climate between 68° and 78°
  - Fuel capacity no less than 175 miles
  - Ground clearance of at least 6" from ground
  - Able to perform at temps from –30°F to 122°F
  - Clearly marked with name of service no less than 3" high and identified from sides and rear of ambulance

Lights and Sirens
- Must be equipped with a siren capable of emitting sounds audible under normal conditions from 500 feet
- Must have at least one light capable of displaying a red light with 360° capacity (or strobe lights) that are visible under normal conditions from 500 feet

Road Hazards/Mechanical Failure
- Must be minimally equipped with:

- Flashlight
- Road marking device
- Tools, wrench, screwdriver, hammer
- Leather, heavy-duty gloves
- Reflective vests
- Equipment with dealing with snow as appropriate to the environment

Communications Equipment
- Radio frequencies must adhere to state EMS radio communication plans
- Must have a PA-system with output of 45 watts
- There must be means of communication other than a cell phone:
    - Between driver and patient compartments
    - Surface vehicle and medical control
    - Surface vehicle and public safety agencies

CAMTS Radio Standards
- Radio transmissions must be able to transmit to/from:
    - Medical direction
    - Communication center
    - Air traffic control and other aircraft
    - Emergency services responding to scenes with the aircraft

Inclement Weather Policy
- There must be a written policy addressing weather and environmental conditions that prohibit transport in conditions of zero visibility and/or official road closures

No More "Ambulance Drivers"
- The driver must be at a minimum certified as an EMT
- The driver must have 2 years of experience as a licensed driver
- The driver must have completed defensive driving & an approved EVOC
- There must be a "co-pilot"

Maintenance Standards
- Preventative maintenance program required and completed by a certified mechanic/shop specific for the make and model of the vehicle
- There must be no evidence of damage penetrating the body or holes that may allow exhaust to enter the patient compartment
- The interior must be kept clean and aligned with OSHA standards
- Must be daily vehicle checks documented
- Fluid and tire pressure checks twice a week

QUESTIONS:

1. You have sustained a hard landing and the pilot is unconscious. What is the best course of action to turn off the aircraft?

    a. Kill engines
    b. Kill battery
    c. Pull rotor break
    d. Meet at 6 o'clock position

2. Which of the following is NOT pertinent information when deciding to accept a flight request?

    a. Acuity of patient
    b. Geography
    c. Weather
    d. IFR vs. VFR

Chapter 9 citations:

1. Rexford Penn Group. (2013). Crew Resource Management: A Guide for Professional Pilots. (1)*******
2. https://www.faa.gov/regulations_policies/handbooks_manuals/aviation/helicopter_flying_handbook/media/hfh_ch11.pdf (2)**
3. Maresh, Woodrow, Webb. (2016). Handbook of Aerospace and Operational Physiology, 2nd Ed. USAF: Wright-Patterson AFB.
4. (3)**
5. https://www.faasafety.gov/files/gslac/library/documents/2013/mar/75375/nvgs2.pdf (4)****
6. https://www.faa.gov/news/safety_briefing/2016/media/SE_Topic_16-12.pdf (5)***
7. https://www.camts.org/wp-content/uploads/2017/06/Safety-Culture-Survey.pdf
8. (6)***
9. https://www.aviationmedicine.com/article/smoking-cessation-and-tobacco-abuse/ (7)***
10. https://www.camts.org/wp-content/uploads/2017/05/CAMTS-11th-Standards-DIGITAL-FREE.pdf (8)
11. https://www.safekidswi.org/Safe-Kids/Documents/Technician-Support-Documents/SafePediatricTransportinAmbulances.pdf (9)
12. https://www.camts.org/wp-content/uploads/2017/05/2018-Special-Ops-standards.pdf (10)
13. https://www.faa.gov/about/initiatives/lasers/laws (11)
14. CAMTS. Eleventh Edition Accreditation Standards.

CHAPTER 10: CARDIOLOGY

PART ONE: Cardiac Conditions

CARDIAC ANATOMY & PHYSIOLOGY

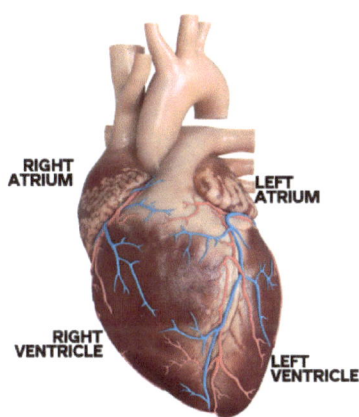

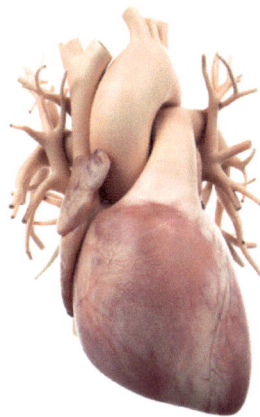

ANTERIOR VIEW   POSTERIOR VIEW   CROSS SECTION

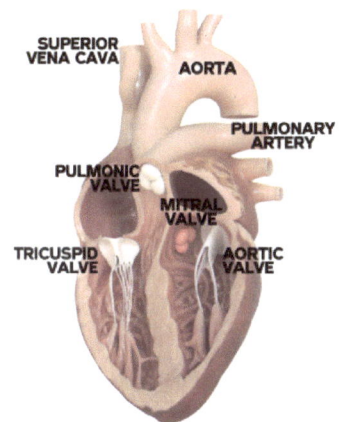

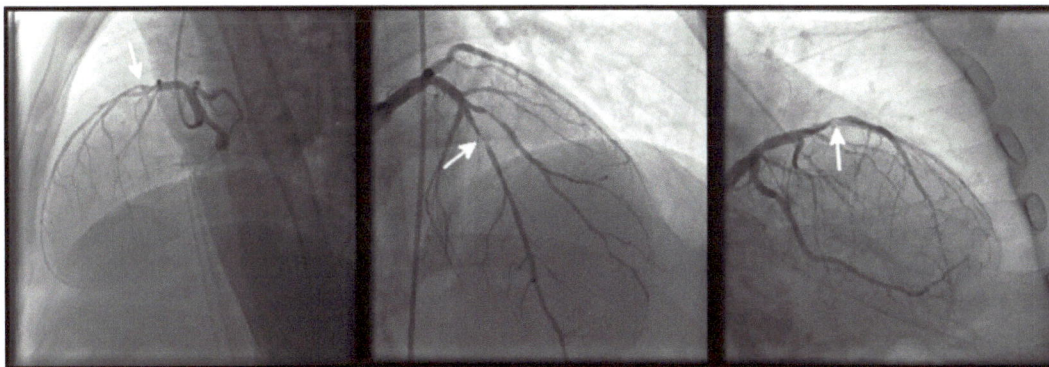

THE FIRST THING THAT THE HEART PERFUSES IS ITSELF VIA THE CORONARY ARTERIES.

Heart Valves[1]
- Prevent regurgitation
- Mitral: left
- Tricuspid: right
- Semilunar valves
  - Pulmonic
  - Aortic

CARDIAC OUTPUT[1] = HEART RATE x STROKE VOLUME
Normal Value: 4-8 L/min

Preload is the amount of blood returning to the heart.

Ejection Fraction is a volumetric representation of stroke volume.
Normal Value: 60-65%

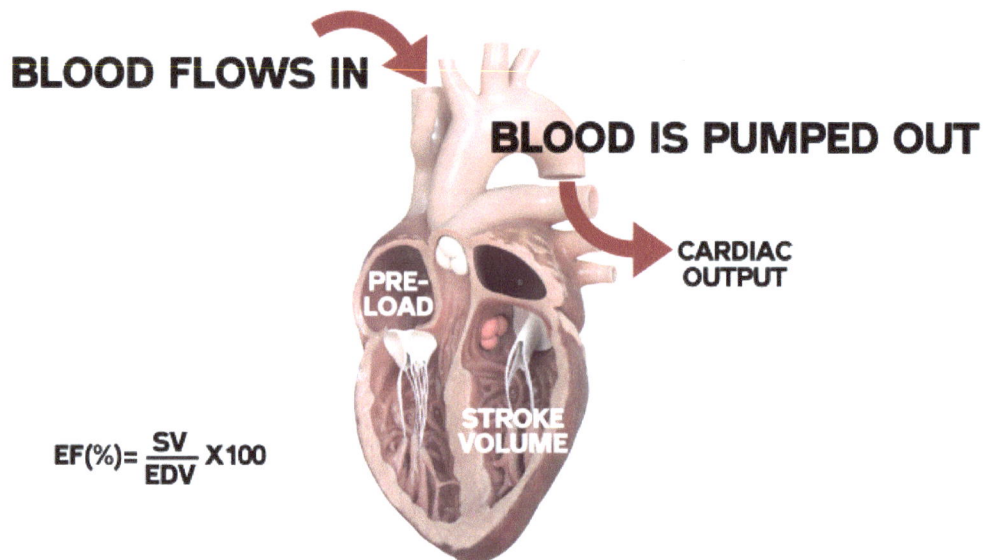

$$EF(\%)= \frac{SV}{EDV} \times 100$$

AFTERLOAD is the resistance against which the Left Ventricle has to pump against to get blood out of the heart. Afterload is affected by Systemic Vascular Resistance (SVR).

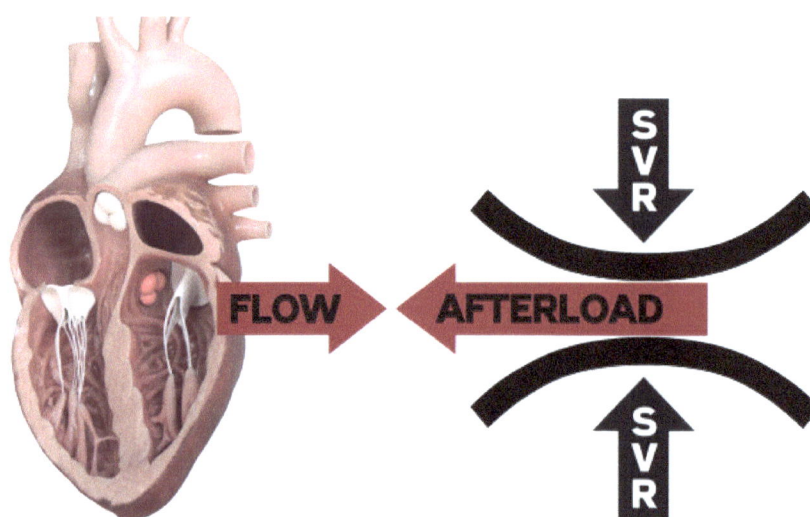

Heart Sounds[1]
S1: Tricuspid & mitral valve closure
S2: Pulmonic & aortic valve closure
S3: Rapid filling of ventricle
S4: Atrial contraction

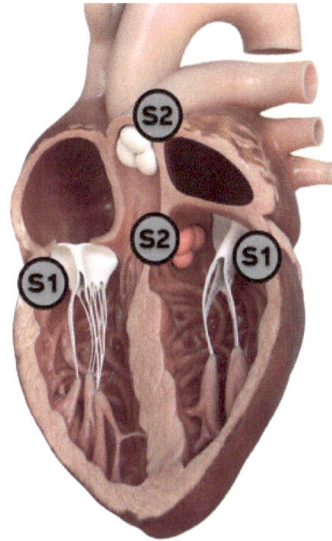

The Electrical Conduction System:

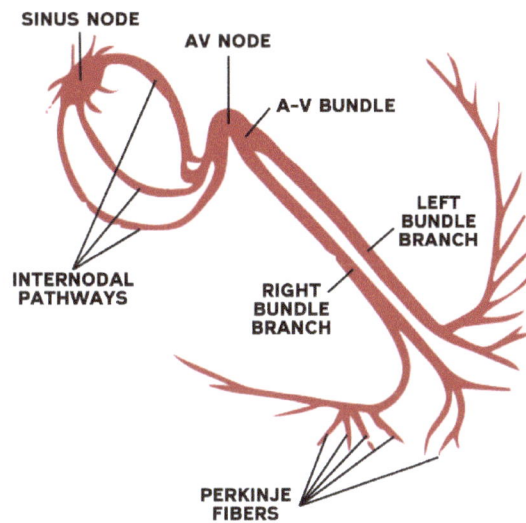

EINTHOVEN'S TRIANGLE

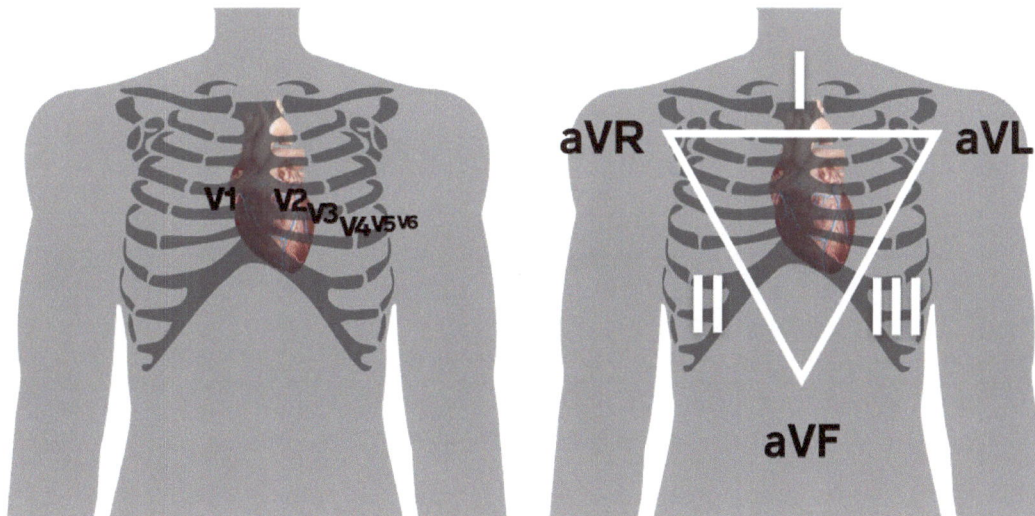

EKG INTERPRETATION

Steps for Every Interpretation:
- **Rhythm**
- **Regularity**
- **Rate**
- **P-wave: is there one for every QRS? Are there extra?**
- **PR interval duration**
- **QRS complex duration and appearance**

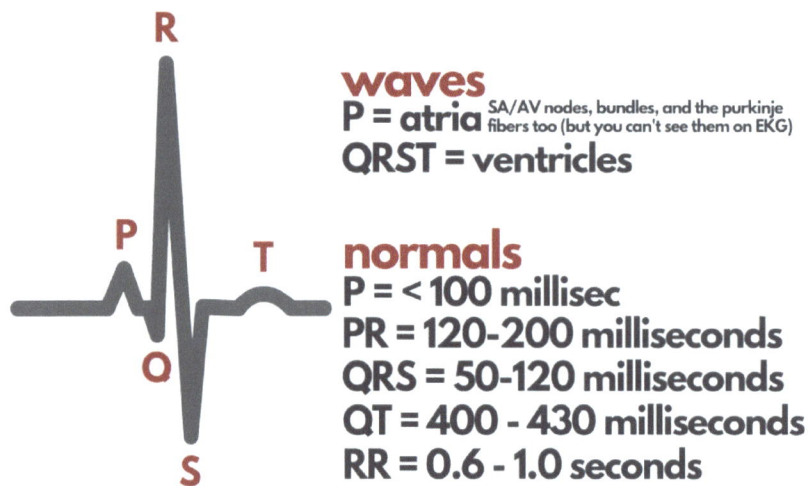

waves
P = atria SA/AV nodes, bundles, and the purkinje fibers too (but you can't see them on EKG)
QRST = ventricles

normals
P = < 100 millisec
PR = 120-200 milliseconds
QRS = 50-120 milliseconds
QT = 400 - 430 milliseconds
RR = 0.6 - 1.0 seconds

COMPONENTS OF THE QRS COMPLEX

P Wave[19]
- Upright: I, II, aVL, and aVF, V5, V6
- Biphasic: III, V1
- Negative deflection: aVR
- Variable: V2, V4

PR Interval (120-200 milliseconds)
- Time between the start of atrial depolarization to the start of ventricular depolarization
  - AV junction is located between atria and ventricles, thus a prolonged PR interval indicates first degree heart block

QRS Complex (50-120 milliseconds)
- Ventricular depolarization
- Electrical signal travels through ventricles via bundle branches

CARDIAC ELECTROLYTES

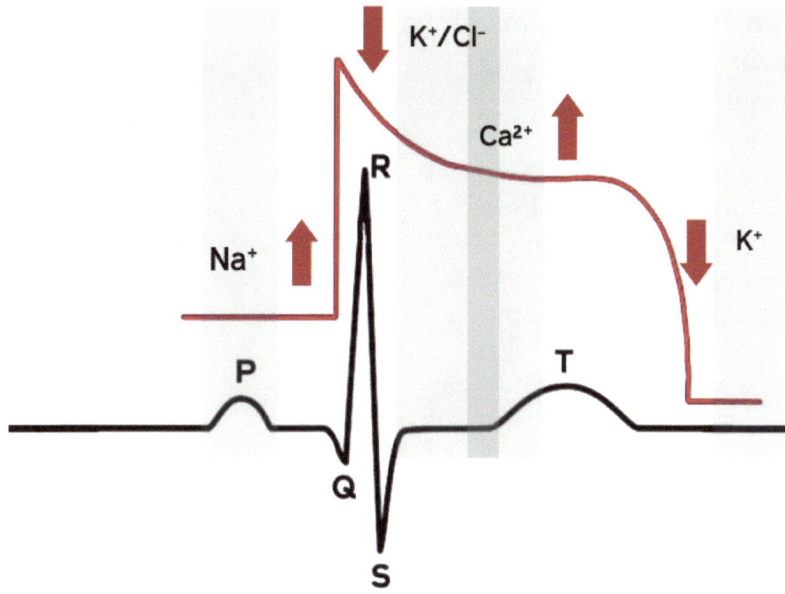

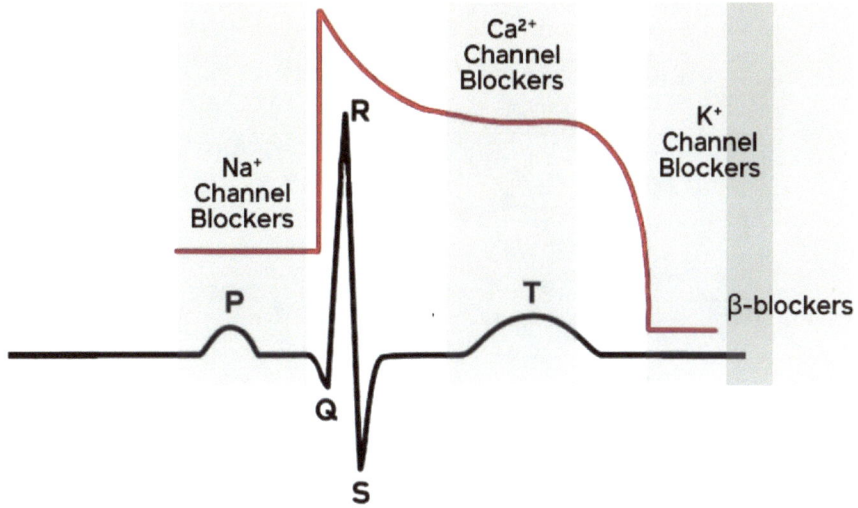

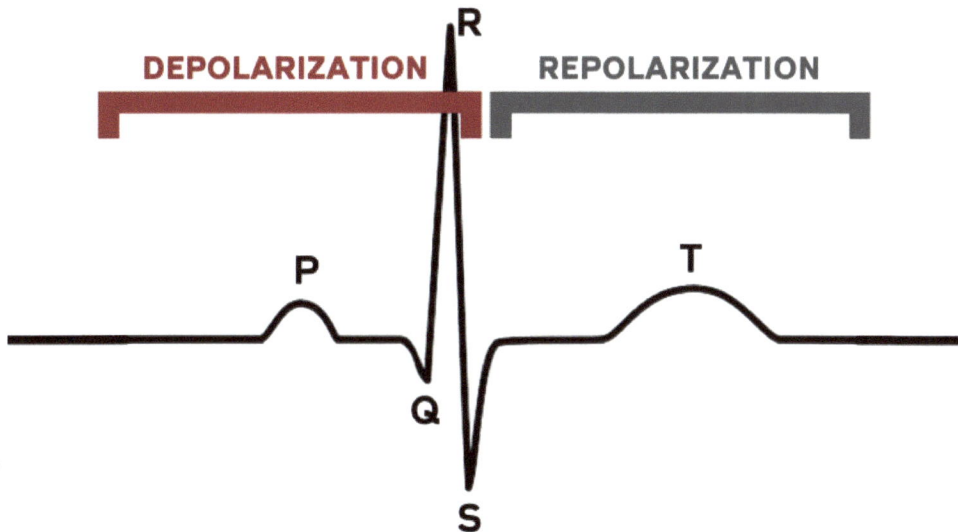

K+/Cl-

Ca²+

Na+

R

P

Q

S

T

Ca²+ Channel Blockers

K+ Channel Blockers

Na+ Channel Blockers

R

P

Q

S

T

β-blockers

DEPOLARIZATION　　　**REPOLARIZATION**

R

P

Q

S

T

AXIS[4,5]

- Represents the sum of all vectors of the ventricles
- Left axis deviation:
  - Often age related
  - Can signify CAD
  - Pregnancy
- Right axis is often normal in kids
- Right axis deviation in adults:
  - Conduction defects
  - Right ventricular strain
  - Helps identify VT

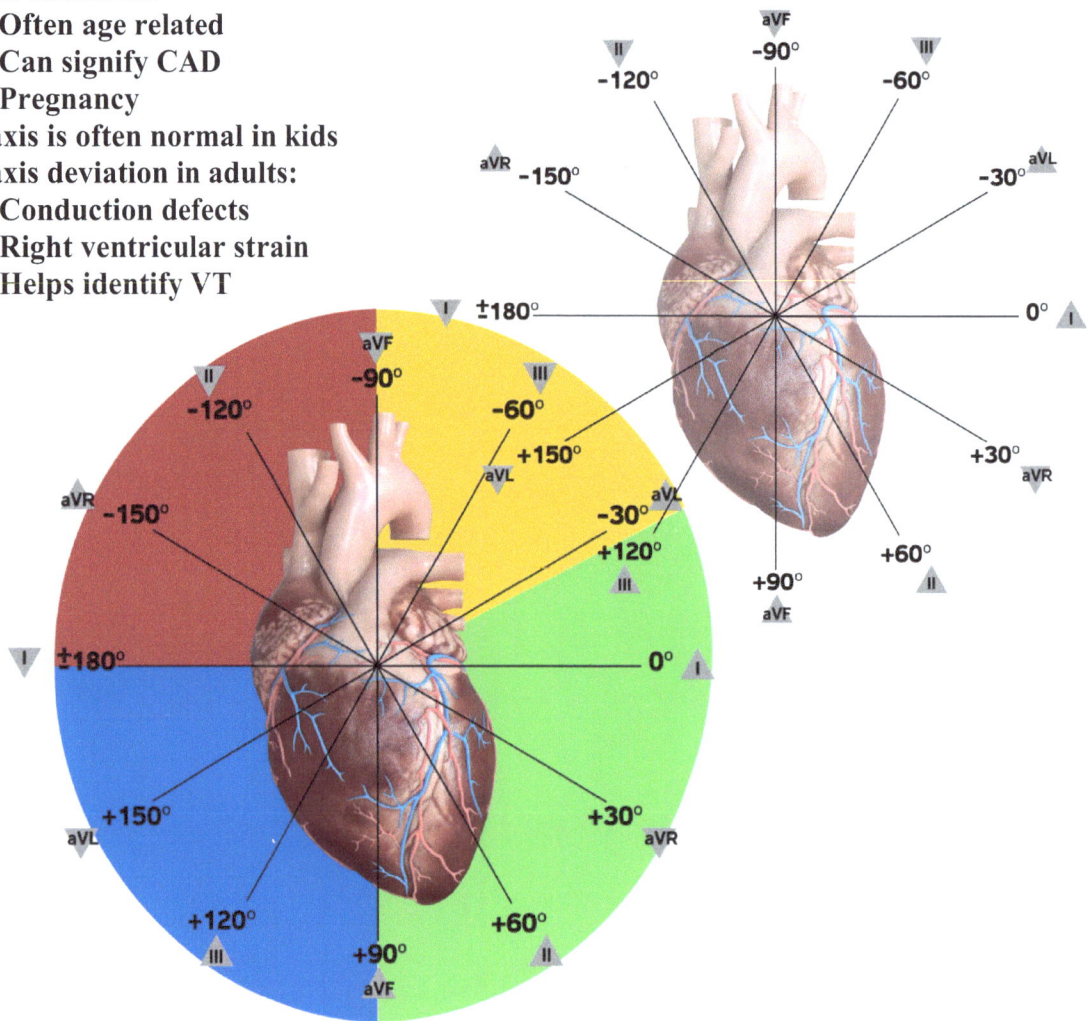

Red: extreme axis deviation, Yellow: left axis deviation, Green: normal, Blue: right axis deviation

ACUTE CORONARY SYNDROME

Angina Pectoris[1]
- **Stable**
  - **Predictable**
  - **Relieved by rest and nitro**
- **Unstable**
  - **Unpredictable onset**
  - **Dynamic presentations**

Myocardial Infarction[10]
- **Death of heart tissue secondary to cessation of blood supply**
- **Type 1: athero-thrombotic event**
- **Type 2: mismatch between O2 supply and demand (ie: stress, coronary vasospasm, shoveling snow)**
- **Type 3: cardiac death with symptoms suggestive of myocardial ischemia and presumed new ischemic ECG changes or new left bundle branch block, but death occurring before blood samples could be obtained**
- **ST Elevation MI[16] (Localization of lesion)**

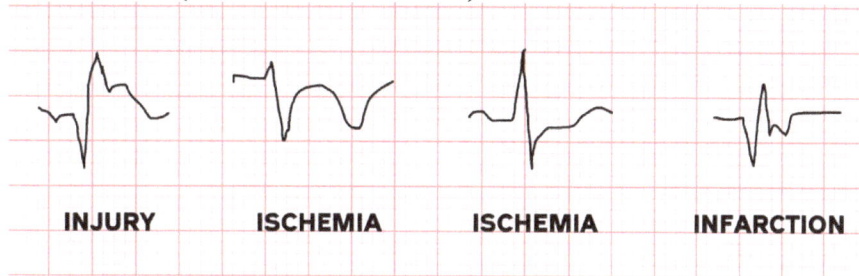

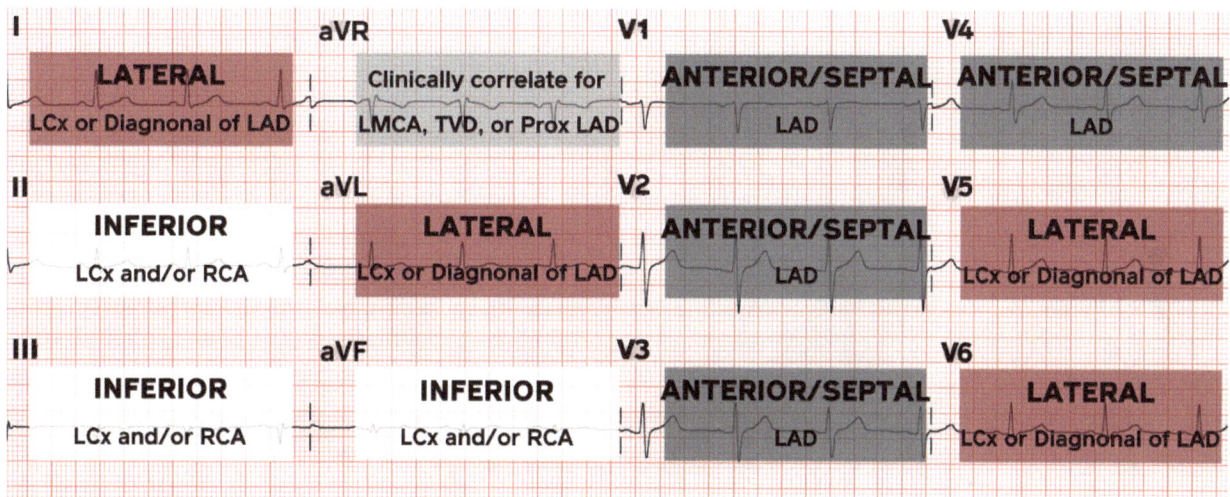

INJURY	ISCHEMIA	ISCHEMIA	INFARCTION

I	aVR	V1	V4
LATERAL LCx or Diagonal of LAD	Clinically correlate for LMCA, TVD, or Prox LAD	**ANTERIOR/SEPTAL** LAD	**ANTERIOR/SEPTAL** LAD
II	aVL	V2	V5
INFERIOR LCx and/or RCA	**LATERAL** LCx or Diagonal of LAD	**ANTERIOR/SEPTAL** LAD	**LATERAL** LCx or Diagonal of LAD
III	aVF	V3	V6
INFERIOR LCx and/or RCA	**INFERIOR** LCx and/or RCA	**ANTERIOR/SEPTAL** LAD	**LATERAL** LCx or Diagonal of LAD

PRO TIP: The patient who is having ACS-like symptoms, has elevation noted in lead aVR, and ischemic changes anywhere else in the 12-lead EKG has a NINETY PERCENT chance of having severe-triple vessel disease!

Inferior Wall MI[10]
- **Involves RCA**
- **High-risk for RV involvement**
  - **Low output heart failure**
  - **Utilize V4R to determine RV involvement**
- **Use nitroglycerin with extreme caution**

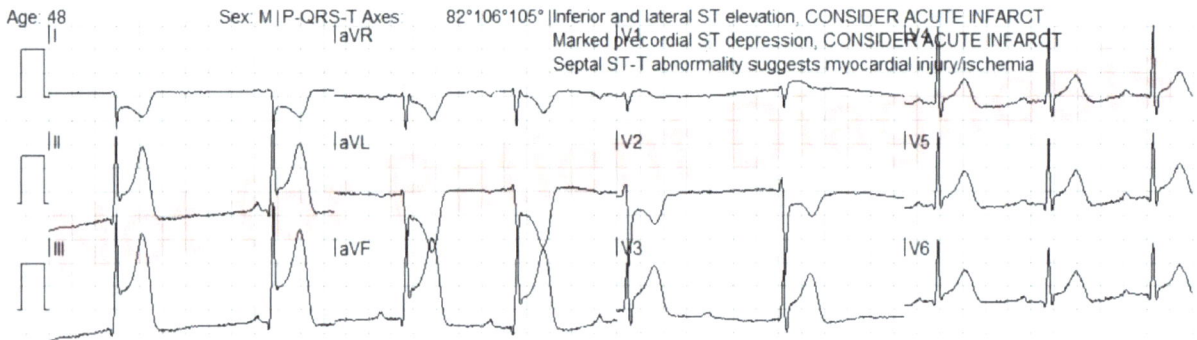

Right sided EKG in Inferior MI:

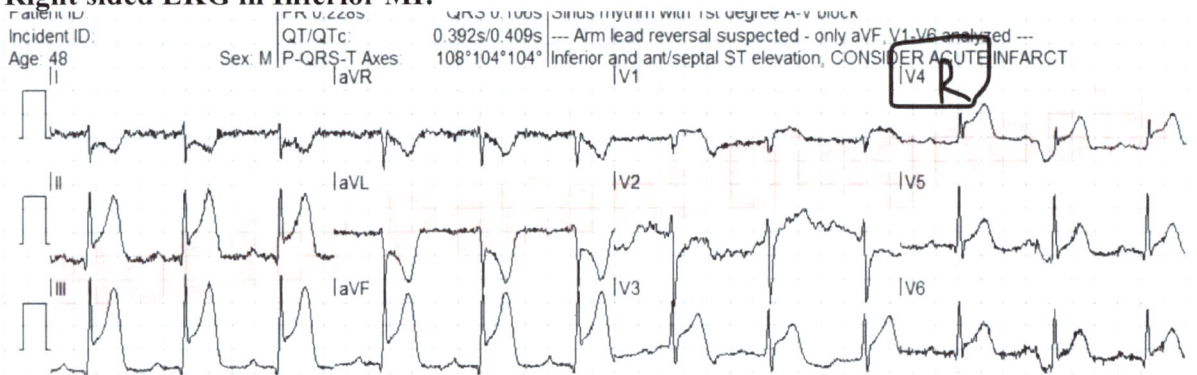

Posterior Wall MI: Large ST depressions in anterior leads (especially V2-V4)

Non-STEMI[10]
- **Does NOT mean less serious**
- **Similar to unstable angina but involves thrombosis**
- **Atypical symptoms in women, elderly, diabetics**

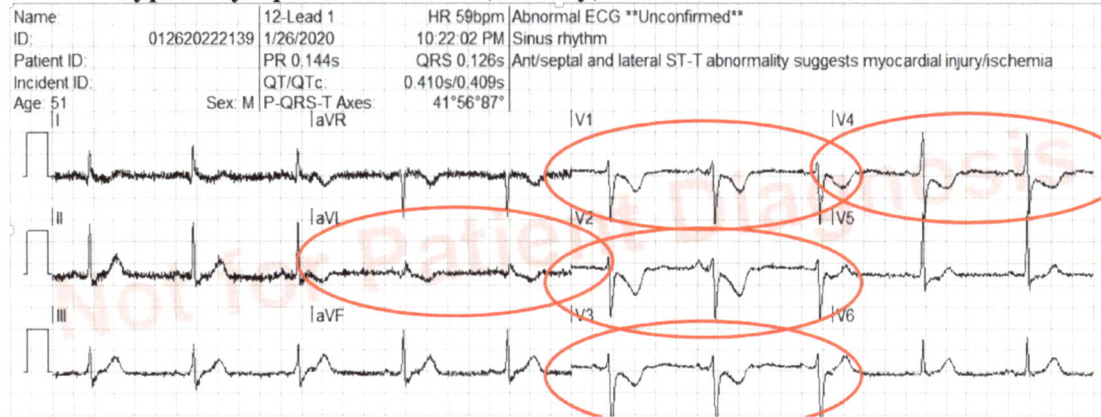

Name:		12-Lead 1		HR 59bpm	Abnormal ECG **Unconfirmed**
ID:	012620222139	1/26/2020		10:22:02 PM	Sinus rhythm
Patient ID:		PR 0.144s		QRS 0.126s	Ant/septal and lateral ST-T abnormality suggests myocardial injury/ischemia
Incident ID:		QT/QTc:		0.410s/0.409s	
Age: 51	Sex: M	P-QRS-T Axes:		41°56°87°	

CARDIAC BIOMARKERS[10]

CKMB and Myoglobin
- **Elevates early**
- **Decreases early**
- **Used to be a standard test**
- **Not specific to cardiac muscle**

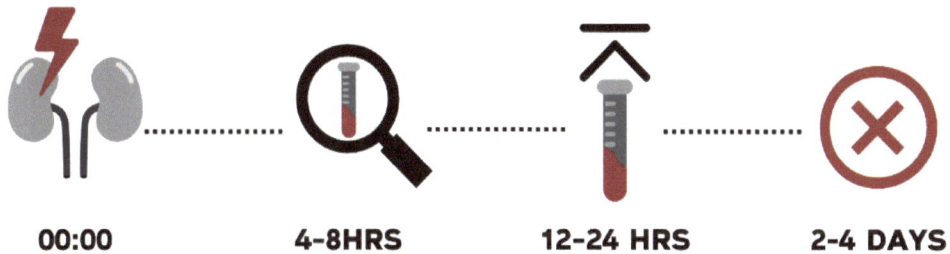

00:00   4-8HRS   12-24 HRS   2-4 DAYS

Troponin
- **Troponin I: Highly cardiac specific**
- **Troponin T: Highly cardiac specific**
- **Troponin C: Not as cardiac specific**

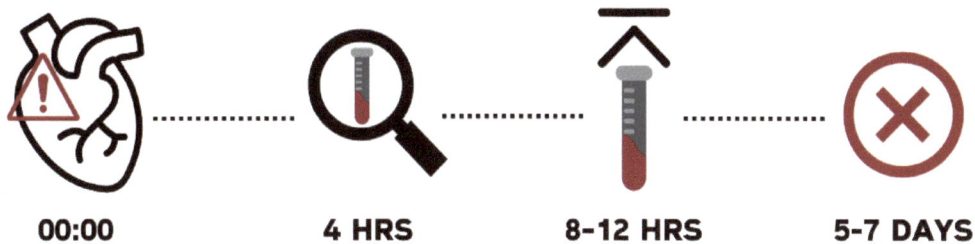

00:00   4 HRS   8-12 HRS   5-7 DAYS

ACS THERAPY

Morphine[6]
- Opiate analgesic
- Histamine release causes vasodilation
- Used to be staple but not anymore
    - EBM: worsens outcomes
    - EBM: associated with more thrombotic events
    - Inhibits ticagrelor (Brilinta)

Nitroglycerin[8,10]
- No reduction in long-term morbidity and mortality
- Possible "short term" reduction in mortality
- Does effectively treat chest pain

Aspirin[9]
- Only ACS drug repeatedly shown to reduce overall all-cause mortality

Beta Blockers[10]
- Mixed data
- Usually not included in prehospital or critical care transport protocols for Acute Coronary Syndrome

Oxygen[7,10]
- No evidence to support routine oxygen administration
- Oxygen is a potent vasoconstrictor

HEART FAILURE

Heart Failure Mechanisms[10]
- Volume overload
- Pressure overload
- Myocardial damage
- Restrictive filling

Starlings Law[10]
- Increased preload causes more myocardial stretch
- Increased stretch of the LV causes more force of contraction

Systolic vs. Diastolic Heart Failure
- Systolic: Reduced Ejection Fraction
- Diastolic: Preserved Ejection Fraction

Brain Natriuretic Peptide[10]
- Activated with myocardial stretch and damage
- Cardioprotective enzyme
- <100: rules out HF
- >500: rules in HF

Right Heart Failure[1]
- Dependent edema
- Organomegaly
- Not life-threatening when chronic right HF
- Causes:
  - Left heart failure (#1)
  - COPD
  - Pulmonary hypertension
  - Pulmonary embolism

Left Heart Failure[1]
- Cause: LV dysfunction
- Pulmonary circuit becomes engorged
- Too much preload
- Increased afterload

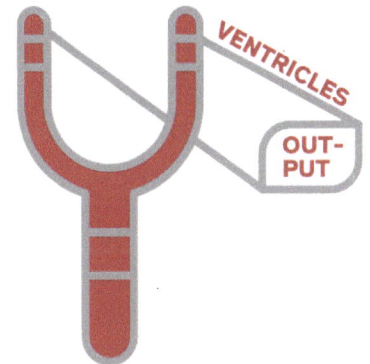

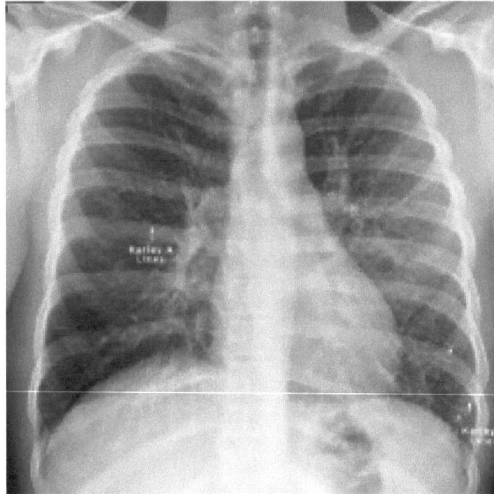

Kerley B-lines in heart failure: Feathery infiltrates moving outward from mediastinum

Acute Decompensated HF[1,10]
- "Flash pulmonary edema"
- 65-75% of HF hospitalizations
- Precipitating factor disrupts CV function
- IV nitroglycerin push (Tridil)
  - Usually 200-400 mcg IV push
  - Standard vasodilator therapy has been shown to not be as effective as IV nitro push in initial stages of acute HF (Gyory, et. al., 2021).

Cardiogenic Shock[1,10]
- Heart cannot pump sufficiently to maintain perfusion
  - Hypotension with hypoperfusion
  - Most common cause is acute MI
- Treatment
  - Inotropes and vasopressors
  - Rapid and judicious fluid challenge
  - Vasodilators contraindicated

Heart Failure Treatment Goals[1,2,10]

- **Restore respiratory function**
- **Optimize fluid volume**
- **Improve hemodynamics**
- **Address underlying cause**

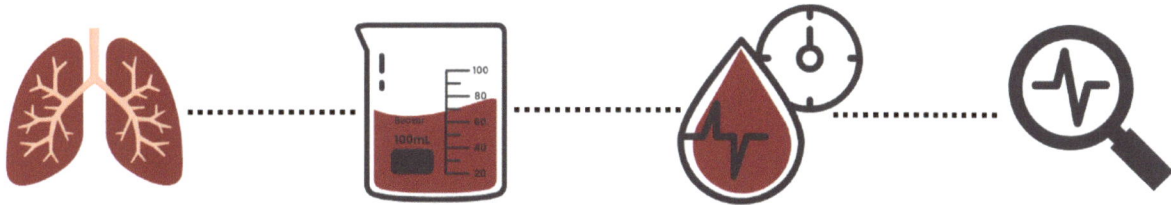

Positive-End Expiratory Pressure[1,2,10]

- **Increases area available for alveolar gas exchange**
- **Equalizes pressure gradient across lungs and pulmonary vasculature**
- **Practice pearl: Coach the patient through NIV**

Nitrates[2,10]

- **Vasodilation relieves pulmonary congestion**
- **Preload reduction**

Loop Diuretics[2,10,11]

- **Recommended for all patients with acute heart failure with signs and symptoms of fluid overload**
- **Diuretics are not commonly in prehospital heart failure protocols**

Positive Inotropy

- **Increases contractility**
- **Indication: cardiogenic shock**
- **NOT a definitive treatment**

Positive Inotropes[10]

- **Dobutamine**
  - **Primary Beta-1 agonist**
  - **Increases cardiac output**
  - **Reduces PCWP**
- **Dopamine**
  - **Beta-1 predominant**
  - **Some Alpha-1 effect**
- **Milrinone**
  - **Phosphodiesterase inhibitor**
  - **Increases inotropy**
  - **Potent vasodilator**
  - **Decreases SVR and PVR**
  - **Reduces filling pressures**

MISCELLANEOUS CARDIAC CONDITIONS

Heart Transplant[13]
- Early dysfunction is quite common
- Heart is denervated:
    - May require pacemaker
    - High intrinsic rate: 90-100
    - Atropine has no effect
    - Increased sensitivity to preload and elasticity

Bundle Branch Block: Look at V1[4]
- >.12 s QRS duration
- Look at first deflection before the J-Point
    - If it is up: RIGHT BBB
    - If it is down: LEFT BBB
- Is this a left or a right BBB?

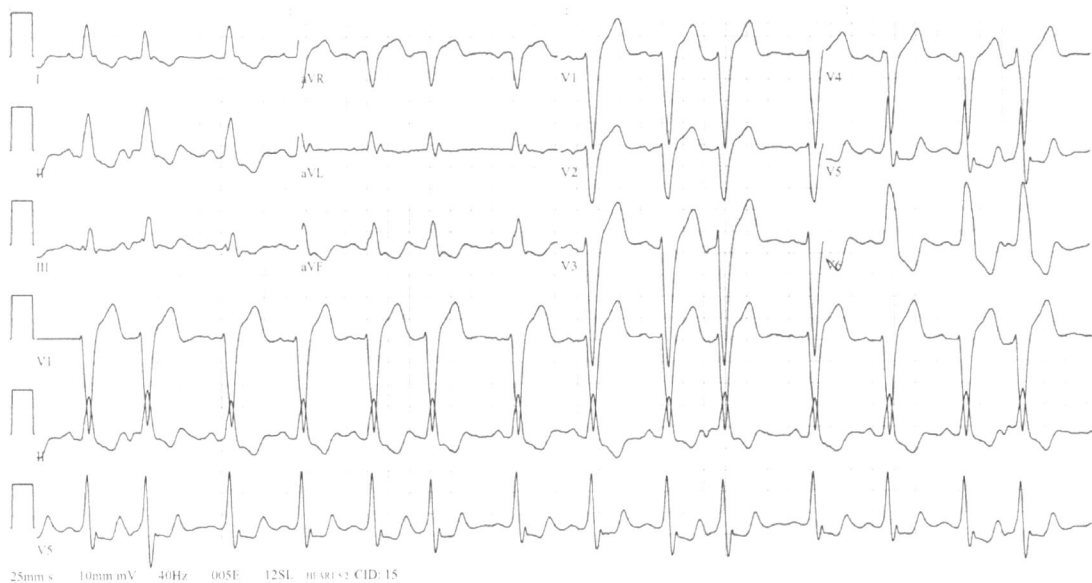

Wolff-Parkinson White[10]

- **Abnormal conduction circuit: Bundle of Kent**
- **Impulse gets trapped: tachyarrhythmias**
- **Verapamil contraindicated**
- **EKG shows "slurred" R wave**

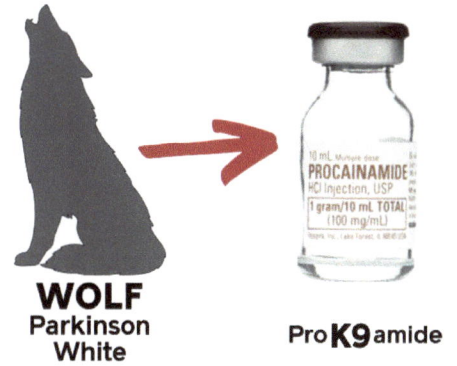

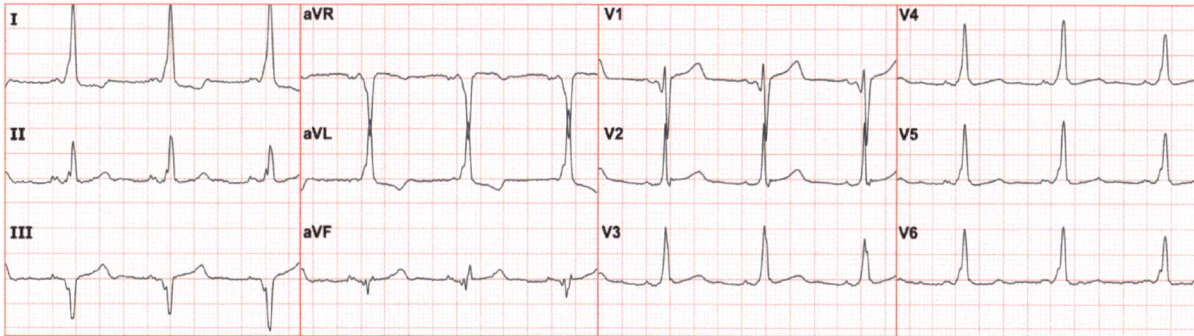

WOLF
Parkinson
White

Pro K9 amide

Atrial Fibrillation[10]

- **Most common sustained arrhythmia in humans**
- **Replacement of P waves by rapid oscillations**
- **Adenosine can help unmask atrial activity (negative dromotrope on AVN)**
- **Anti-coagulation if > 48 hours**

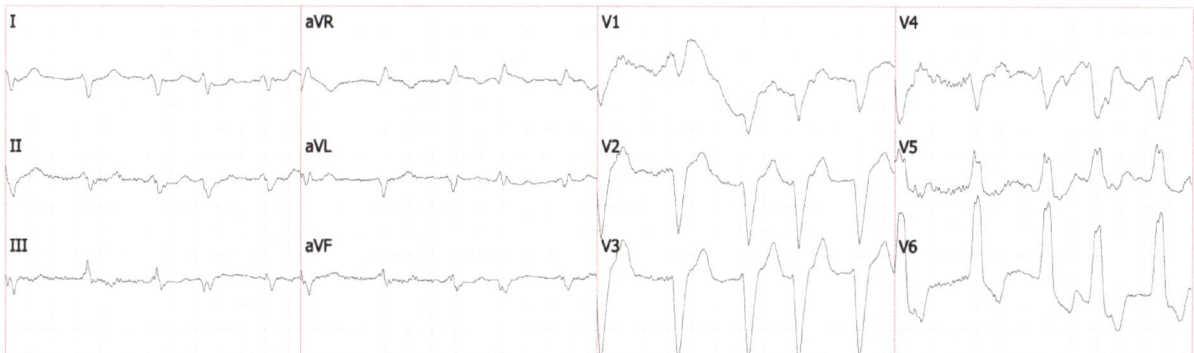

Supraventricular Tachycardia

- **HR >150 bpm, re-entry phenomenon**
- **Stable: adenosine, vagal maneuvers**
- **Unstable: synchronized cardioversion**

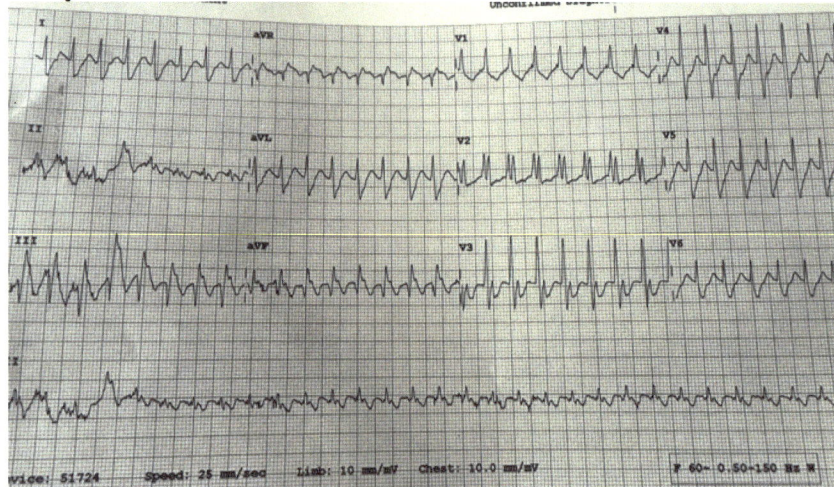

Ventricular Tachycardia

- **70-80% of wide-complex tachycardia is VT**
- **Precordial negativity concordance**
- **When in doubt, treat as VT**

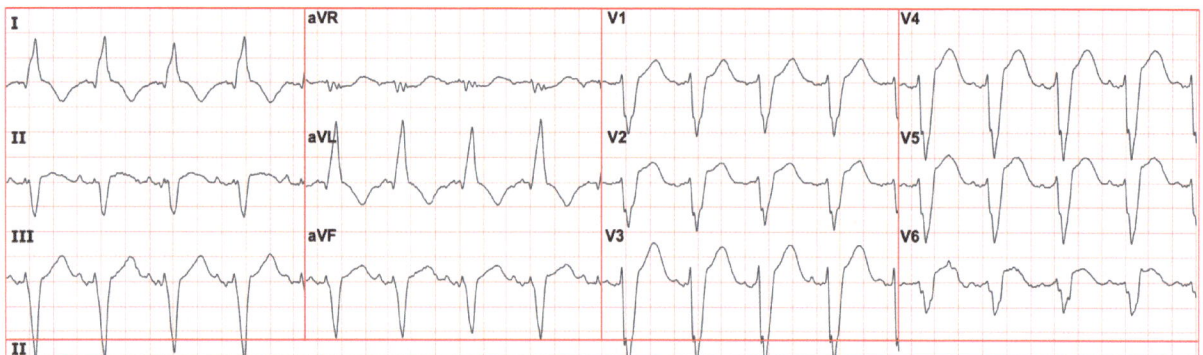

Myocarditis[10]

- **Wide-ranging presentation and severity**
  - **Chest pain**
  - **Heart failure**
  - **Arrhythmia**
- **Fever present in most cases**
- **High risk of ventricular arrhythmias**
- **Risk of dilated cardiomyopathy**

Pericarditis[10]
- Pleuritic chest pain
- Pain worse with inspiration and supine positioning
    - Patients will prefer pronation, leaning forward, etc.
- Flu-like symptoms may precede onset

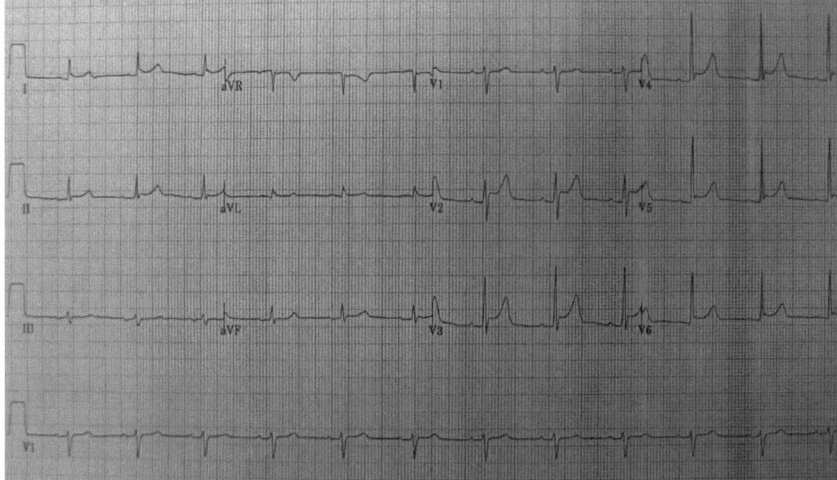

Endocarditis[3,10]
- Surgical emergency
- Risk factors
    - Valve replacement, IV drug use, dialysis
- Presentation
    - Fever and malaise
    - Septic shock
    - Heart failure from valve regurgitation
    - Septic emboli

Endocarditis Exam Findings[10]
- Fever
- New murmur
- Splinter hemorrhages
- Conjunctival hemorrhages
- Janeway Lesions
- Osler Nodes

AORTIC EMERGENCIES

Aortic Dissection[10]
- Long-term hypertension is number one risk factor
- Risk with connective tissue disorders
- 85% diagnosed after death
- 40% die immediately

Dissection Presentation[10]
- Often presents as "tearing" or "ripping" pain
- Back pain suggests Type B
- Chest pain suggests Type A
- Often tachycardic and hypertensive

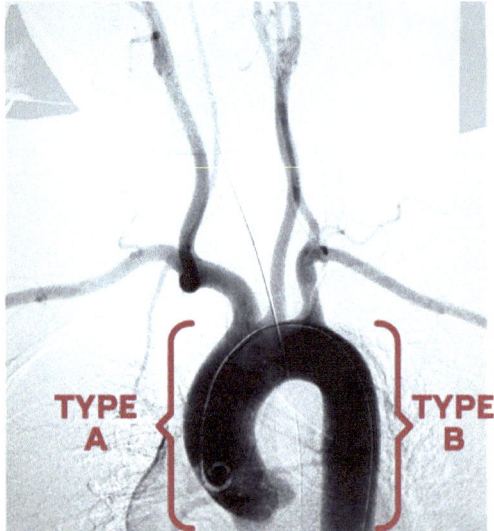

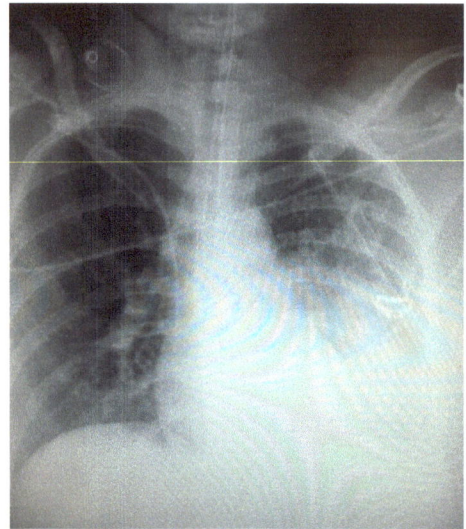

Chest X-Ray
- Widened mediastinum
- Abnormal aortic knob
- Maybe left pleural effusion

Dissection Treatment[10]
- Anti-impulse therapy is priority
- HR goal: 60-70 bpm
- SBP goal: <120 mmHg
- Aggressive analgesia

Abdominal Aortic Aneurysm[14]
- Majority are asymptomatic
- Classic rupture presentation:
  - Severe abdominal pain
  - Hypotension
  - Pulsatile mass
- Transport goal is to "keep them alive"
- Treatment: immediate surgical repair

Chapter 10: PART 1 CITATIONS:

1. American Academy of Orthopaedic Surgeons (AAOS). (2022). Critical Care Transport Navigate Essentials Access (3rd ed.). Jones & Bartlett Learning.

2. Colucci, W. (2022). Treatment of Acute Decompensated Heart Failure. Up-to-Date.

3. Farkas, J. (2021, July 4). Endocarditis. EMCrit.org. https://emcrit.org/ibcc/endo/

4. Goldberger, A. (2022). Basic approach to delayed intraventricular conduction. Up To Date.

5. Kashou AH, Basit H, Chhabra L. Electrical Right and Left Axis Deviation. [Updated 2022 Jun 7]. In: StatPearls [Internet]. Treasure Island (FL): StatPearls Publishing; 2022 Jan-. Available from: https://www.ncbi.nlm.nih.gov/books/NBK470532/

6. Salim Rezaie, "The Death of MONA in ACS: Part I – Morphine", REBEL EM blog, November 5, 2017. Available at: https://rebelem.com/the-death-of-mona-in-acs-part-i-morphine/.

7. Salim Rezaie, "The Death of MONA in ACS: Part II – Oxygen", REBEL EM blog, November 5, 2017. Available at: https://rebelem.com/death-mona-acs-part-ii-oxygen/.

8. The Death of MONA in ACS: Part III – Nitroglycerin", REBEL EM blog, November 5, 2017. Available at: https://rebelem.com/death-mona-acs-part-iii-nitroglycerin/.

9. "The Death of MONA in ACS: Part IV – Aspirin", REBEL EM blog, November 5, 2017. Available at: https://rebelem.com/death-mona-acs-part-iv-aspirin/.

10. Tubaro, M., Vranckx, P., Price, S., Vrints, C., & Bonnefoy, E. (2021). The ESC Textbook of Intensive and Acute Cardiovascular Care (The European Society of Cardiology Series) (3rd ed.). Oxford University Press.

11. Pan, A., Stiell, I. G., Dionne, R., & Maloney, J. (2015). Prehospital use of furosemide for the treatment of heart failure. Emergency medicine journal : EMJ, 32(1), 36–43. https://doi.org/10.1136/emermed-2013-202874

12. De Backer, D., Biston, P., Devriendt, J., Madl, C., Chochrad, D., Aldecoa, C., Brasseur, A., Defrance, P., Gottignies, P., & Vincent, J. L. (2010). Comparison of Dopamine and Norepinephrine in the Treatment of Shock. New England Journal of Medicine, 362(9), 779–789. https://doi.org/10.1056/nejmoa0907118

13. Gerlach, R. (2022). Anesthesia for Heart Transplantation. Up-to-Date.

14. Dalman, R., & Mell, M. (2022b). Overview of abdominal aortic aneurysm. Up to Date.

15. Thompson, B. T., & Kabrhel, C. (2022). Overview of acute pulmonary embolism in adults. Up to Date.

16. Akbar H, Foth C, Kahloon RA, et al. Acute ST Elevation Myocardial Infarction. [Updated 2022 Aug 1]. In: StatPearls [Internet]. Treasure Island (FL): StatPearls Publishing; 2022 Jan-. Available from: https://www.ncbi.nlm.nih.gov/books/NBK532281/

17. EMCrit, A., & Farkas, J. (2021, November 29). Submassive & Massive PE. EMCrit Project. https://emcrit.org/ibcc/pe/

PART TWO: HEMODYNAMIC MONITORING

Arterial Monitoring[1,2]
- Invasive, continuous, real-time BP monitoring
- Provides numeric and waveform display of the patient's cardiovascular status
- Achieved through cannulation of a peripheral artery

The Arterial Waveform:

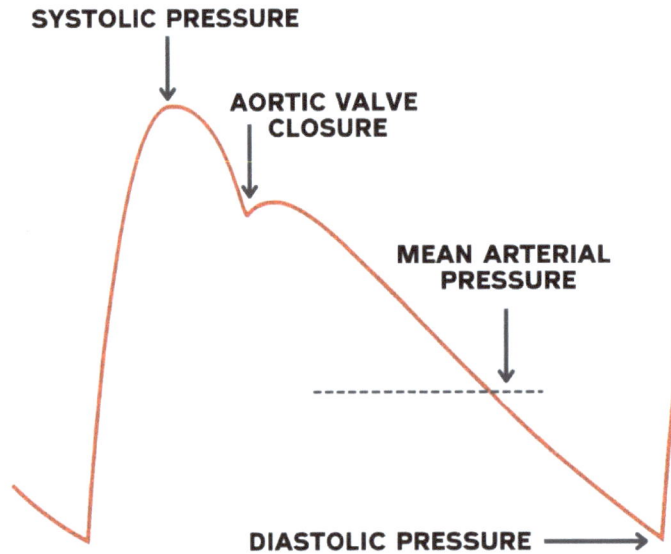

Arterial Line Set Up:

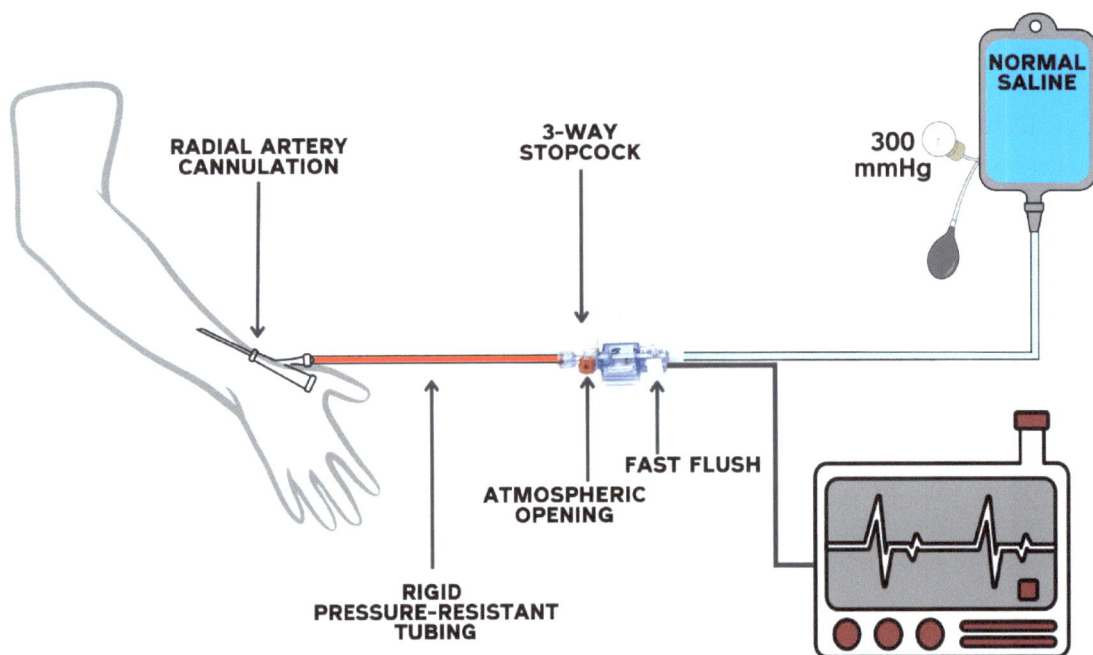

Transducer:
- Phlebostatic axis: 4th ICS anterior mid-axillary line
- Zero when transitioning between monitors and with significant altitude change

Zeroing the Line[1,3,4]

- **Ensures accurate measurements**
- **Zeroing provides a "zero reference pressure" according to atmospheric pressure**

1. TRANSDUCER AT PHLEBOSTATIC AXIS

2. STOPCOCK OFF TO PATIENT

3. REMOVE CAP FROM ATMOSPHERIC OPENING

4. PRESS "ZERO" BUTTON ON MONITOR

5. CAP ATMOSPHERIC OPENING

6. OPEN STOPCOCK TO TRANSDUCER

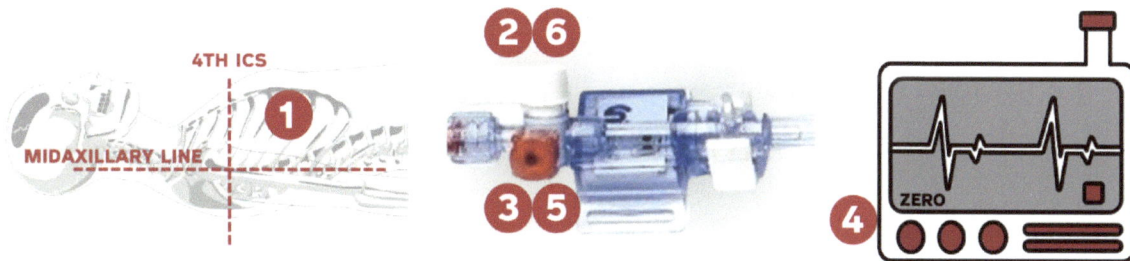

Fast Flush Test[4]

Three oscillations post fast flush when appropriately transduced

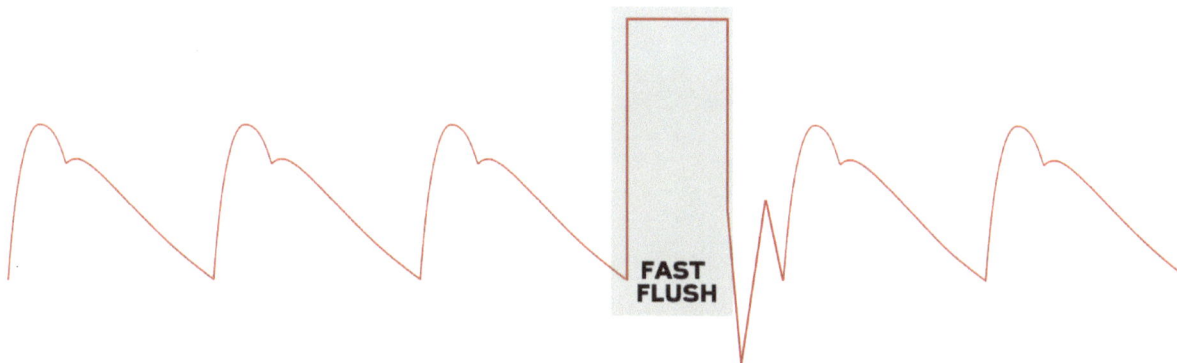

FAST FLUSH

Overdampening[1,4]

- **Will yield a falsely low systolic BP**
- **May be due to a clot on the catheter tip, air bubbles, kinks in line**

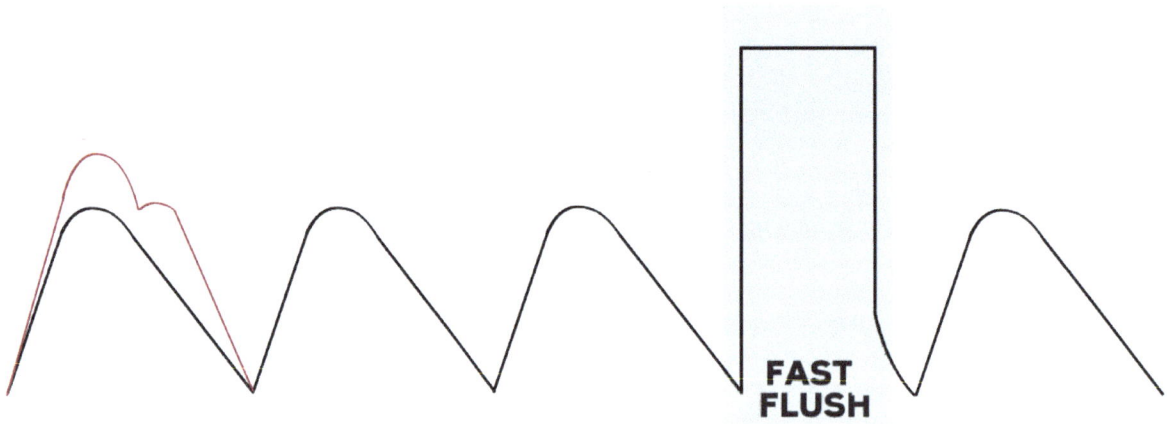

Underdampening[1,4]

- **Overestimation of systolic BP and underestimation of the diastolic BP**
- **Due to catheter whip, low pressure on fluids bag, tachydysrhythmias**

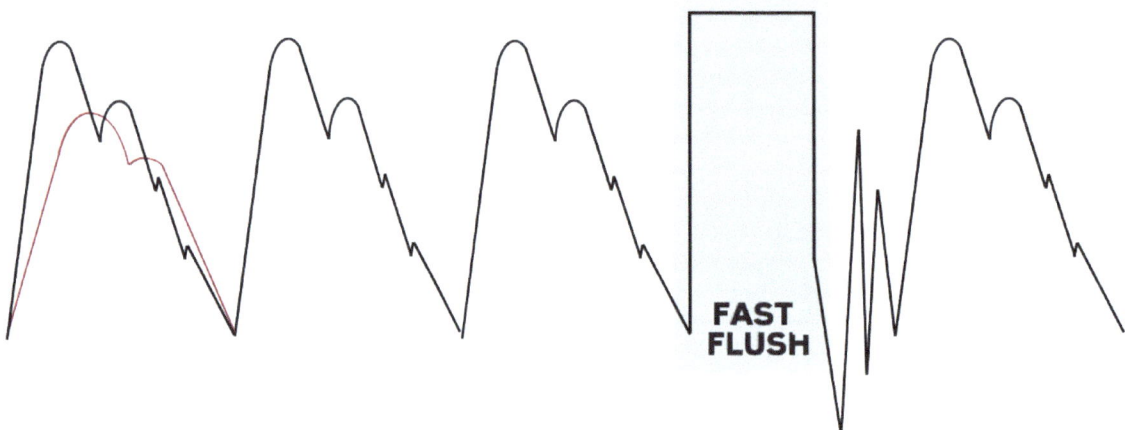

Cordis Line[5]

- **Large central venous access catheter**
- **Preferred central line for any situation where rapid infusion is anticipated**
- **Short, wide, single-lumen**

Pulmonary Artery Catheter (aka: Swan-Ganz)[6,7,8]

- **Provides numerous hemodynamic and oxygen delivery data points**
- **Threaded through vena cava, through right-side of heart, and into pulmonary artery**
  - **If it migrates into RV, PULL BACK DO NOT ADVANCE**
- **Most frequently used in cardiac ICU settings**

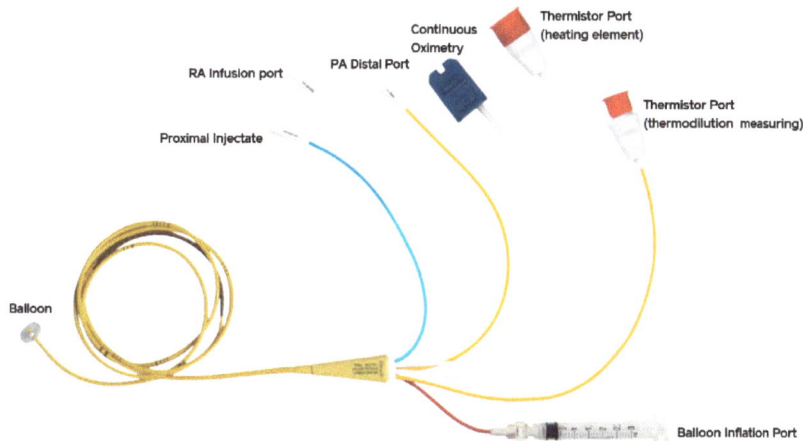

- **Balloon port is red: PASSIVELY deflate balloon, 1.5mL capacity**
- **Must be deflated during transport, NEVER wedge in transport**
- **Transduce yellow port**

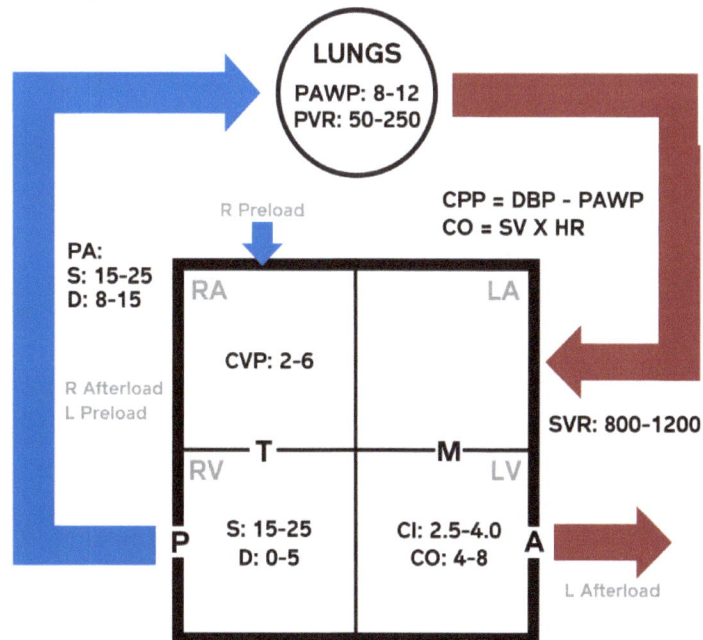

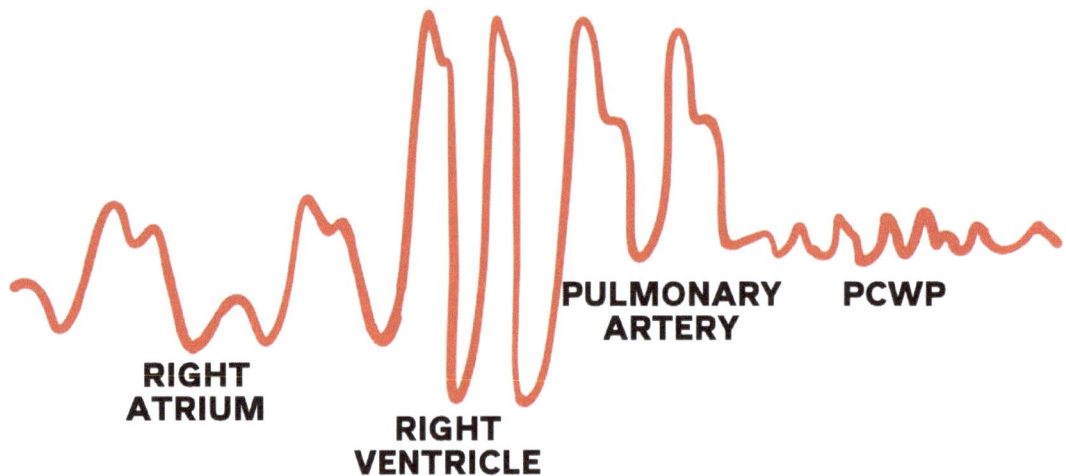

RIGHT ATRIUM **RIGHT VENTRICLE** **PULMONARY ARTERY** **PCWP**

RA Waveforms[6,7]
- Measures central venous pressure (CVP)
- Normal CVP: 2-6 mmHg

RV Waveform[6,7,8]
- Great risk of arrhythmia
- Ensure the balloon is deflated
- Gently withdraw until a RA waveform appears
- Normal pressure values:
  - 15-25 mmHg systolic
  - 0-5 mmHg diastolic

PA Waveform[6,7]
- This is what you want to see during transport
- Normal PA pressures:
  - 15-25 systolic
  - 8-15 diastolic

Pulmonary Artery Wedge Pressure[6,7]
- Displays atrial systole and atrial diastole (filling)
- Used to measure left heart preload
- If elevated, indicates INCREASED PRELOAD
- It is BRIEFLY measured (no more than 3 patient breath cycles)
- Normal value: 8-12 mmHg

Mixed Venous Oxyhemoglobin Saturation (SvO$_2$)[9]
- Measures the oxygen content of the blood returning to the right side of the heart
- Normal SvO$_2$: 65-70%
- When O$_2$ supply does not meet the metabolic demands, SvO2 will be abnormal
- Increased SvO$_2$: increased O$_2$ delivery, decreased demand
- Decreased SvO$_2$: elevated O$_2$ consumption/demand

PA Cath: Indirect Measurements[7]
- Systemic vascular resistance
- Pulmonary vascular resistance
- Cardiac Index
- Stroke volume index
- LV stroke work index
- RV stroke work index
- Oxygen Delivery
- Oxygen Uptake

Cardiac Index[7]
- Reflects cardiac function in relation to the patient's size
- CI = CO/BSA
- Normal values: 2.5-5.0 L/min/m^2

Systemic Vascular Resistance[7]
- SVR = [(MAP – right atrial pressure)/CO] x 80
- Normal SVR: 800-1200 dyne
- High SVR: Vasoconstriction
- Low SVR: Vasodilation

Pulmonary Vascular Resistance[7]
- Most often elevated in pulmonary hypertension

Oxygen Delivery and Consumption[10]
- DO$_2$: The rate at which oxygen is delivered to the microcirculation from the lungs
- VO$_2$: The rate at which oxygen is removed from the blood by the tissues
- Fick principle at work

The "RiCH ANSwer" to Invasive Cardiology

	TYPE OF SHOCK	SVR 800-1200	C.I 2.5-5.0	CVP 2-7	PAWP 8-12
Ri	RVMI	HIGH	LOW	HIGH	LOW
C	CARDIOGENIC	HIGH	LOW	HIGH	HIGH
H	HYPOVOLEMIC	HIGH	LOW	LOW	LOW
A	ANAPHYLACTIC	LOW	LOW	LOW	
N	NEUROGENIC	LOW	LOW		
S	SEPTIC	LOW	HIGH		

Original source unknown

SVR: RiCH high, ANS low
CI: All low except last
CVP: RiCH- ANSwer is 2 words, 2 HIGH, 2 LOW
PAWP: Low-High-Low

Chapter 10: Part 2 citations:

1. Nguyen Y, Bora V. Arterial Pressure Monitoring. [Updated 2022 Sep 18]. In: StatPearls [Internet]. Treasure Island (FL): StatPearls Publishing; 2022 Jan-Available from: https://www.ncbi.nlm.nih.gov/books/NBK556127/

2. Weiner R, & Ryan E, & Yohannes-Tomicich J (). Arterial line monitoring and placement. Oropello J.M., & Pastores S.M., & Kvetan V(Eds.), Critical Care. McGraw Hill. https://accessanesthesiology.mhmedical.com/content.aspx?bookid=1944&sectionid=143522170

3. Esper, S. A., & Pinsky, M. R. (2014). Arterial waveform analysis. Best practice & research. Clinical anesthesiology, 28(4), 363–380. https://doi.org/10.1016/j.bpa.2014.08.002

4. "Damping and Arterial Lines", REBEL EM blog, July 4, 2022. Available at: https://rebelem.com/damping-and-arterial-lines/.

5. Pologe, J. (2018, August 27). Cordis Placement POD. Maimonides Emergency Medicine. https://www.maimonidesem.org/blog/cordis-placement-pod

6. Edwards Life Sciences Corp. (2018). Swan-Ganz Pulmonary Artery Catheter. Available: http://Edwards.com/clinicaleducation

7. Fleitman, J. (2022). Pulmonary artery catheterization: Interpretation of hemodynamic values and waveforms in adults. Up-to-Date.

8. Weinhouse, G. (2022). Pulmonary Artery Catheters: Insertion Techniques in Adults. Up-to-Date.

9. Shanmukhappa, S., & Lokeshwaran, S. (n.d.). Venous Oxygen Saturation. National Library of Medicine. https://www.ncbi.nlm.nih.gov/books/NBK564395/

10. Rosen, I., & Manaker, S. (2022). Oxygen Delivery and Consumption. Up to Date.

Part Three: Mechanical Circulatory Support

Mechanical Circulatory Support[2]
- Usually used as a "bridge to decision"
- Goal
  - Increase myocardial oxygen supply and reduce demand
  - Biggest risk
  - Thromboembolism

Intra-Aortic Balloon Pump (IABP)[2]
- Relatively simple
- Cost effective
- DOES NOT provide direct cardiac support
- DOES NOT provide flow

IABP Indications[2,4]
- Adjunct treatment in high risk PCI
- MI with decreased ventricular function
- Low cardiac output state after CABG
- Bridge to treatment in patients with any of the following conditions:
  - Intractable angina
  - Refractory myocardial ischemia
  - Refractory heart failure***
  - Refractory ventricular arrhythmias

IABP Contraindications[2,4]
- Severe aortic valve insufficiency
- Severe aortic regurgitation
- Severe peripheral artery disease
- Acute aortic dissection

Counterpulsation[2]
- Balloon inflates in diastole: perfuses coronary arteries
- Balloon deflates in systole: reducing afterload
- 24% increase in cardiac index
- 31% reduction in myocardial afterload

IABP Trigger[4]
- Two triggers
  - EKG
  - Arterial Waveform (pressure)

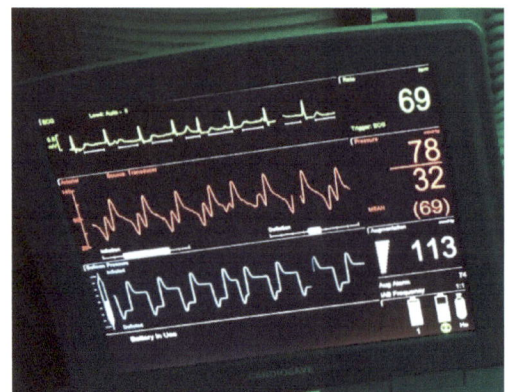

IABP TIMING AND WAVEFORMS

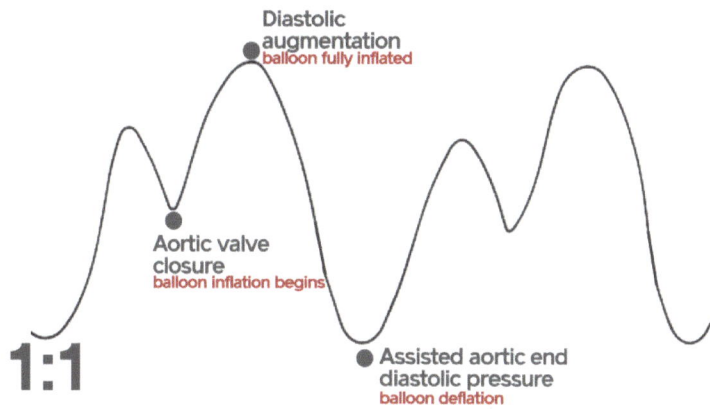

1:1

Diastolic augmentation
balloon fully inflated

Aortic valve closure
balloon inflation begins

Assisted aortic end diastolic pressure
balloon deflation

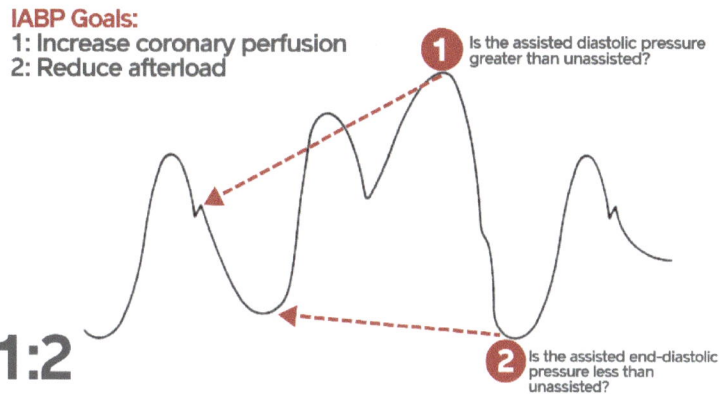

IABP Goals:
1: Increase coronary perfusion
2: Reduce afterload

1:2

1 — Is the assisted diastolic pressure greater than unassisted?

2 — Is the assisted end-diastolic pressure less than unassisted?

Checking for Timing Errors:
- **Must be in 1:2 or 1:3 timing to compare with unassisted pressures**

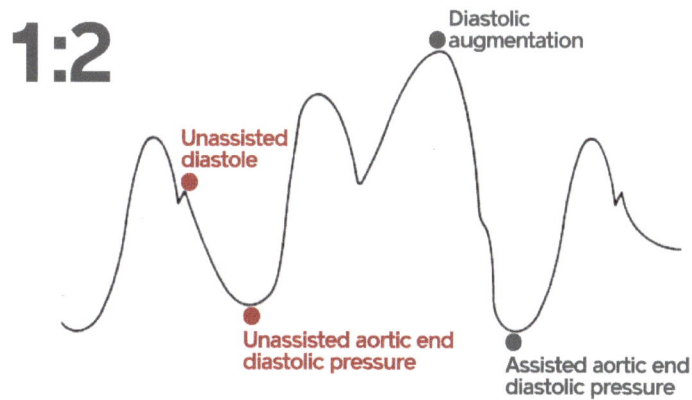

1:2

Diastolic augmentation

Unassisted diastole

Unassisted aortic end diastolic pressure

Assisted aortic end diastolic pressure

IABP timing error: EARLY INFLATION

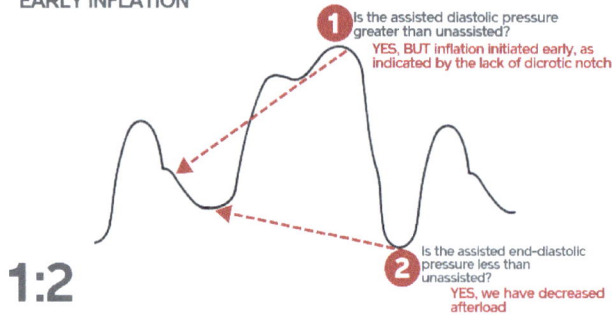

1 Is the assisted diastolic pressure greater than unassisted?
YES, BUT inflation initiated early, as indicated by the lack of dicrotic notch

2 Is the assisted end-diastolic pressure less than unassisted?
YES, we have decreased afterload

1:2

IABP timing error: LATE INFLATION

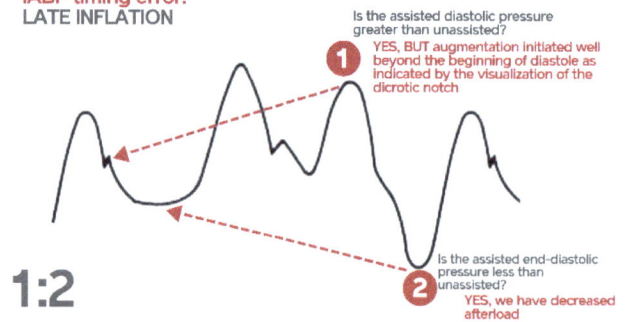

1 Is the assisted diastolic pressure greater than unassisted?
YES, BUT augmentation initiated well beyond the beginning of diastole as indicated by the visualization of the dicrotic notch

2 Is the assisted end-diastolic pressure less than unassisted?
YES, we have decreased afterload

1:2

IABP timing error: EARLY DEFLATION

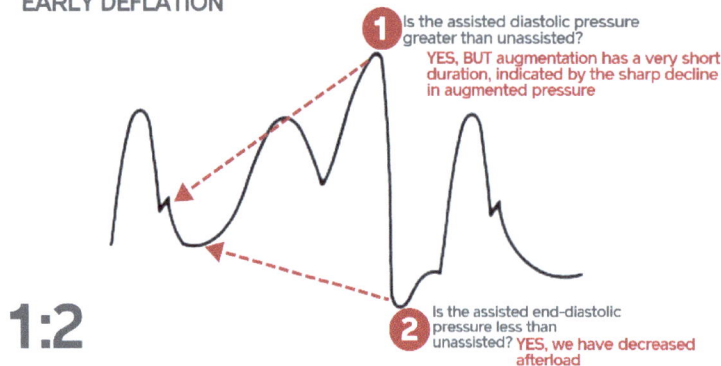

1 Is the assisted diastolic pressure greater than unassisted?
YES, BUT augmentation has a very short duration, indicated by the sharp decline in augmented pressure

2 Is the assisted end-diastolic pressure less than unassisted? YES, we have decreased afterload

1:2

IABP timing error: LATE DEFLATION

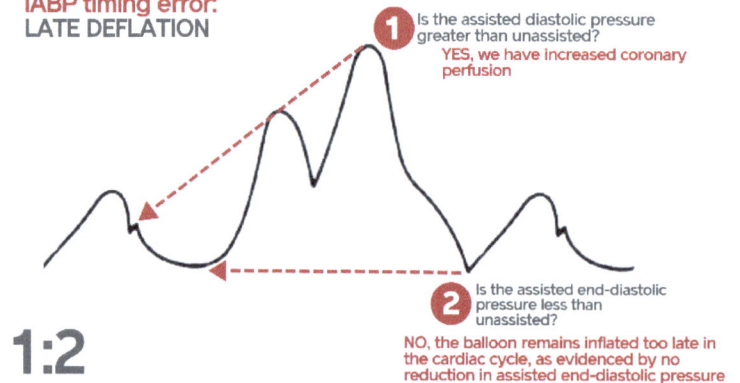

1 Is the assisted diastolic pressure greater than unassisted?
YES, we have increased coronary perfusion

2 Is the assisted end-diastolic pressure less than unassisted?
NO, the balloon remains inflated too late in the cardiac cycle, as evidenced by no reduction in assisted end-diastolic pressure

1:2

IABP Complications[2]
- Site bleeding (1.4%)
- Vascular injury (0.7%)
- Major limb injury (0.5%)
- Amputation (0.1%)
- Bowel, renal, spine infarcts (0.1%)

Impella[2,3]
- Short-term assist device
- Pumps blood directly into aorta
- Pumping from LV is most common
- May also be used in:
  - Left atrium
  - Right ventricle (temporarily)

Left Ventricular Assist Device[1]
- Indication: advanced heart failure
- Primary Goal: prolong survival and improve quality of life
- May be used as bridge to transplant
- Increases perfusion and reduces filling pressures of the heart
- Augments heart, does not replace native function entirely

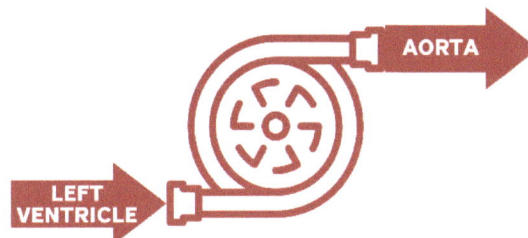

Extra-Corporeal Membrane Oxygenation (ECMO)[2,3]
- Incorporates a centrifugal pump and a membrane oxygenator
- Pulls blood out of the body and into the ECMO machine
- Can be used for up to 30 days
- Optimal functioning is still preload dependent

Venous-Arterial ECMO (V-A)[2]
- Provides hemodynamic support
- Provides flow
- Offloads work of the heart

Venous-Venous ECMO (V-V)[2]
- Indication: refractory respiratory failure
- Does not provide hemodynamic flow support

ECMO Transport Considerations
- Critically ill patient
- Additional staff needed
  - Perfusionist
  - CV surgeon
- Space for equipment, room to work
- Unconventional vent settings
- Patients are prone to hypothermia

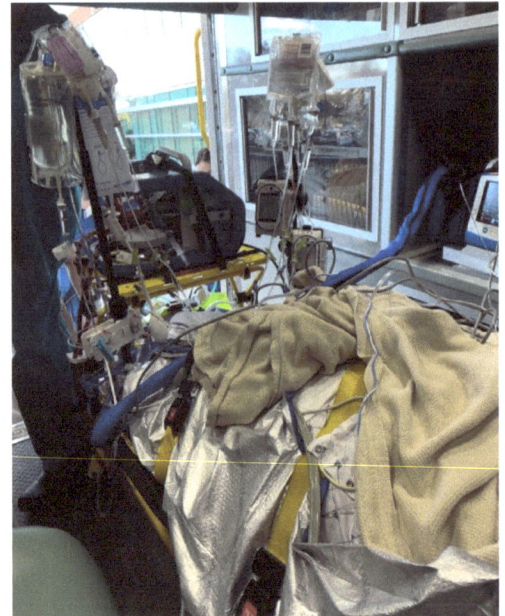

QUESTIONS:

1. The patient presents with malaise and fever. Assessment shows spotty lesions on his palms. A murmur is noted on auscultation of heart tones. Which condition do you suspect?

    a. Myocarditis
    b. Endocarditis
    c. Pericarditis
    d. Oomphycytitis

2. Which of the following occurs during diastole when the patient is receiving IABP support?

    a. The balloon deflates, reducing afterload
    b. The balloon inflates, perfusing the coronaries
    c. The balloon inflates, reducing afterload
    d. The balloon deflates, perfusing the coronaries

Chapter 10: Part 3 citations:

1. Birks, E. J., & Mancini, D. (2022). Treatment of advanced heart failure with a durable mechanical circulatory support device. Up to Date.
2. Tubaro, M., Vranckx, P., Price, S., Prints, C., & Bonnefoy, E. (n.d.). The ESC Textbook of Intensive and Acute Cardiovascular Care (The European Society of Cardiology Series) (3rd ed.). Oxford University Press. p. 355
3. Jeevanandam, V., & Eisen, H. (n.d.). Short-Term Mechanical Circulatory Assist Devices. Up to Date.
4. Khan TM, Siddiqui AH. Intra-Aortic Balloon Pump. [Updated 2022 Jun 3]. In: StatPearls [Internet]. Treasure Island (FL): StatPearls Publishing; 2022 Jan-. Available from: https://www.ncbi.nlm.nih.gov/books/NBK542233/

Chapter 11: Professional Considerations

Just Culture[5]
- Safety supportive system of shared accountability in which health care organizations are accountable for:
  - Systems in place
  - Responding to the actions of their staff in a just manner
- Abandons previous practice of blame assignment
  - Paradigm shift from punitive culture and reprimanded actions toward clinicians to system improvement

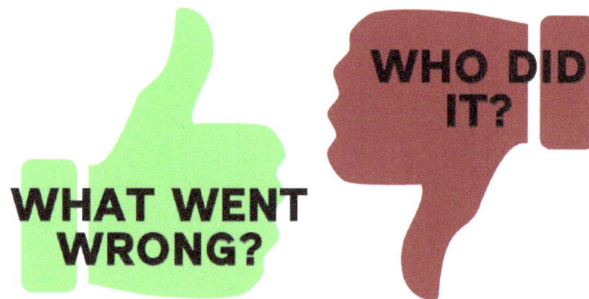

WHAT WENT WRONG?

WHO DID IT?

JUST CULTURE:

a system of shared accountability in which all contributing factors to accidents or sentinel events are considered

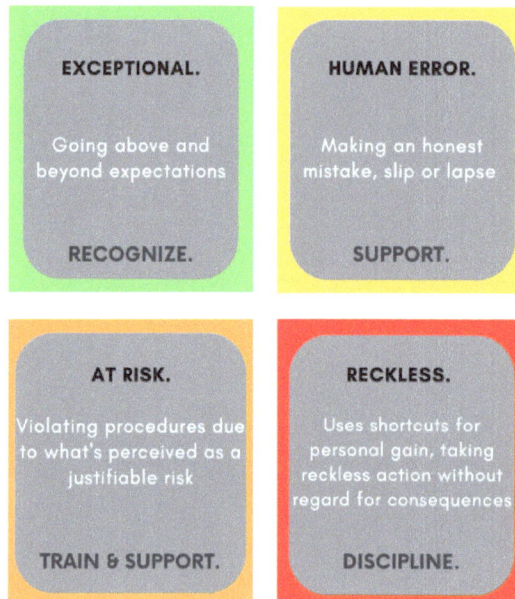

EXCEPTIONAL. Going above and beyond expectations **RECOGNIZE.**	**HUMAN ERROR.** Making an honest mistake, slip or lapse **SUPPORT.**
AT RISK. Violating procedures due to what's perceived as a justifiable risk **TRAIN & SUPPORT.**	**RECKLESS.** Uses shortcuts for personal gain, taking reckless action without regard for consequences **DISCIPLINE.**

Accreditation Standards[1]
- Standards must be maintained to be CAMTS accredited
  - Educational requirements for crew, ethical standards, business profiles, standardization of equipment, crew credentials, safety/weather plans, and maintenance.
- Purpose: ensure safe operations and maximize crew effectiveness
  - CAMTS standards are revised every 2-3 years
  - Accreditation is valid for 3 years

CAMTS Accreditation
- Most common crew configuration in US HEMS is RN (CFRN®) and Paramedic (FP-C)
  - RN/RN
  - RN/MD
  - RNC-OB/ Neonatologist or Neonatal RRT
  - Crew members can include pilot, nurse, paramedic, APRN/PA, physician, or respiratory therapist
  - EMT is not recognized as air crew member

Ground Air Medical Quality Transport (GAMUT) Metrics
- Data analytics platform for medical transport programs to track, report, and evaluate performance on transport-specific quality metrics[2]
  - Airway management
  - Administration of blood products
  - Ventilator management
  - CPR
  - HROB events
  - Safety events

Privacy Considerations[6]
- HIPAA: Health Insurance Portability Accountability Act
  - A 1996 law that created a standard of privacy thresholds healthcare workers must follow
  - Disclose PHI only for TPO purposes
    - Treatment
    - Payment
    - Operations
- What to do?
  - Media: Defer to contact public information officer (PIO)
  - DO NOT post on social media
    - Identifiable or specific information
    - Scene photos or location
    - News articles
  - Do not use personal devices to take pictures or capture PHI
  - Always log off or cover PHI in public settings

Holistic Patient Care

Sedation and Analgesia
- Paralyzed patients experience pain
  - Vital signs
  - Tearing of the eyes
  - Ventilator dyssynchrony as paralytic wears off

Communicating with the Patient
- Auditory senses are the last to fade
  - Verbalize plan of care with all patients, even if unresponsive
  - Use this to help you with care
    - "Can you please swallow?" can help advance a stuck ETT

Death Notification
- OHCA results in death 90% of the time[3]
- Shared understanding in first response community[4]
  - Death is routine
  - Confidence deficit in making death notifications
  - Absence of training in death communication

Grief
- Natural response to loss
- Denial, Anger, Bargaining, Depression, Acceptance
- 3 types of grief
  - Anticipatory
  - Complicated
  - Disenfranchised

Communication During Resuscitation[4]
- 20 minutes on scene with OHCA often portrays the image that may worry, or strike confusion with family members
- "Communication was identified as one of the top risk factors associated with complaints and malpractice allegations"- Alex Jabr
  - In the eyes of the family, provider communication and building rapport with patient's family outweighs how the provider performs clinically
- Prior to transporting a critically ill patient
  - Assure family members and communicate plan of care
  - Share pertinent details of transport
  - Get phone number

Do Not Resuscitate (DNR)
- DNR is a legal document and end of life request
- On scene with a DNR, find out what patient/family wants
- Provide comfort to the patient's family
  - Be physically present
  - Practice active listening
  - Provide reassurance

MOST/MOLST Form
- Medical Orders for Scope or Treatment
  - Legal Document
- Offers a broad range of medical interventions a patient and family can decide on for emergency situations
- Not mandatory, but often seen in conjunction with DNR
- Should be current with patient's medical conditions

Pediatric Death[4]
- Provider tendency to project emotions onto the scene
  - Fear-based scoop and run
- Separating child from parent is detrimental
  - Studies demonstrate benefit to parents when they are present during resuscitation

Death Notification: EMS Role
- Respond to patient family questions honestly and clarity
  - Use words "dead" or "died"
- Be prepared to repeat yourself, give small doses of information
- Allow them to start their natural process of grieving

"Don't tell them to calm down, it works 0% of the time 100% of the time"
-Alexander Jabr, Emergency Resilience

First Responder Response to Trauma
- Important to connect with someone
  - Professional
  - Partner or trusted peer
  - Don't grieve alone

"When we numb the sadness, we numb the joy. When we numb the pain, we numb the hope. When we numb the depression, we numb out the ability to be happy."
-Alexander Jabr, Emergency Resilience

Stress in the first responder

- Signs of first responder stress
  - Chronic fatigue
  - Irritability
  - Negative attitude
  - Declining health
  - Substance abuse
  - Emotional instability
- Chronic and unrelieved stress leads to burnout

Post-call Debrief

The First Responder
- High frequency of critical incidents in EMS
- Critical incident stress debrief
  - Defuse stress associated with event
  - Provide resources to assist with coping after difficult event
  - Mixed responses within community
  - 24-72 hours post-event
  - Colleagues, professional counselors, clergy

Post-Flight Debrief
- Address safety concerns
  - Plan vs. actual occurrences in flight
- Report incidents
  - Laser strikes
  - Near-misses
  - Unforecasted weather
- Performance review
- End result: improve team dynamics

QUESTION:

1. One of the top risk factors associated with patients and families initiating malpractice claims is:

   a. Inexperienced nursing staff
   b. Length of stay in hospital
   c. Number of providers caring for the patient
   d. Poor communication from medical staff

Chapter 11 citations:

1. CAMTS. (n.d.). https://www.camts.org/
2. Home: GAMUT Ground & Air Medical Quality in Transport. (n.d.). https://www.gamutqi.org/
3. CPR Facts and Stats. (n.d.). cpr.heart.org. https://cpr.heart.org/en/resources/cpr-facts-and-stats
4. Death notifications, Alexander Jabr, Emergency Resilience
5. https://www.ncbi.nlm.nih.gov/pmc/articles/PMC3776518/
6. EMS.gov

Chapter 12: Neurologic emergencies

Neurologic Pathology

Monro-Kellie Doctrine[6]

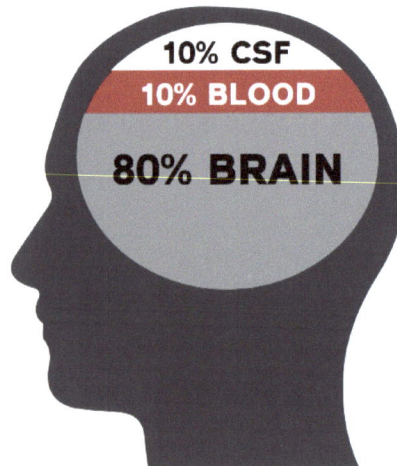

Intracranial Pressure
- **Normal ICP: 5-15 mmHg**
- **Elevated ICP: Cushing's Triad**

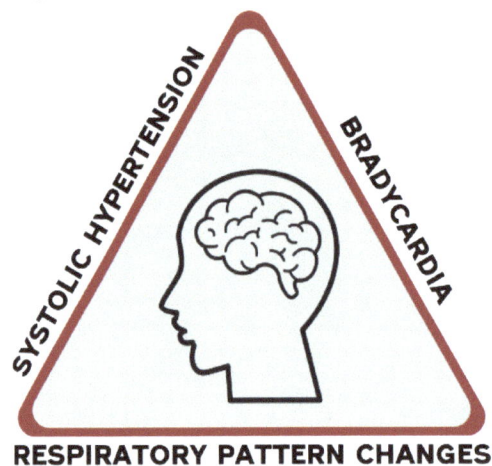

Increased ICP EKG Changes[6]
- **May see ST depressions but most common neuro-related changes are "intracerebral T waves."**
    - **Deep T-waves in anterior leads**

Herniation[6]

- **Risk if ICP is >20 for longer than 5 minutes**
- **Multiple types:**
    - **Uncal: posturing, blown pupil**
    - **Subfalcine (cingulate): cerebral artery compression**
    - **Central Tentorial: Diabetes insipidus – tearing of pituitary**
    - **Upwards: bilateral pupil dilation, decerebrate posturing**
    - **Cerebellar (tonsillar): herniation, AMS, resp arrest**

Mean Arterial Pressure

- **MAP = Diastolic + 1/3 (Systolic – Diastolic)**
- **Normal minimum MAP for neuro patients: >80**
- **Absolute minimum for brain perfusion: >60**

Cerebral Perfusion Pressure[6,9]

- **CPP = MAP – ICP**
- **Normal CPP: 50-90, but Brain Trauma Foundation recommends 60-70**

Scenario:

You are transporting a stroke patient status post hemicraniectomy. After a bolus of propofol for sedation the BP is 92/50. The ICP according to the patient's EVD is 14. **What is the CPP and is it adequate?**

Step 1: Calculate MAP
- **MAP = Diastolic + 1/3 (Systolic – Diastolic)**
- **MAP = 50 + 1/3(92-50)**
- **MAP = 50 + 1/3(42)**
- **MAP = 50 + 13.9**
- **MAP = 64**

Step 2: CPP = MAP – ICP
- **CPP = 64-14**
- **CPP = 50**

Indications for ICP Monitoring
- **Severe TBI**
- **Comatose patients with abnormal CT scan**
- **Hydrocephalus with elevated ICP**
- **Any patient with an anticipated long course of stay where ICP will be a concern**

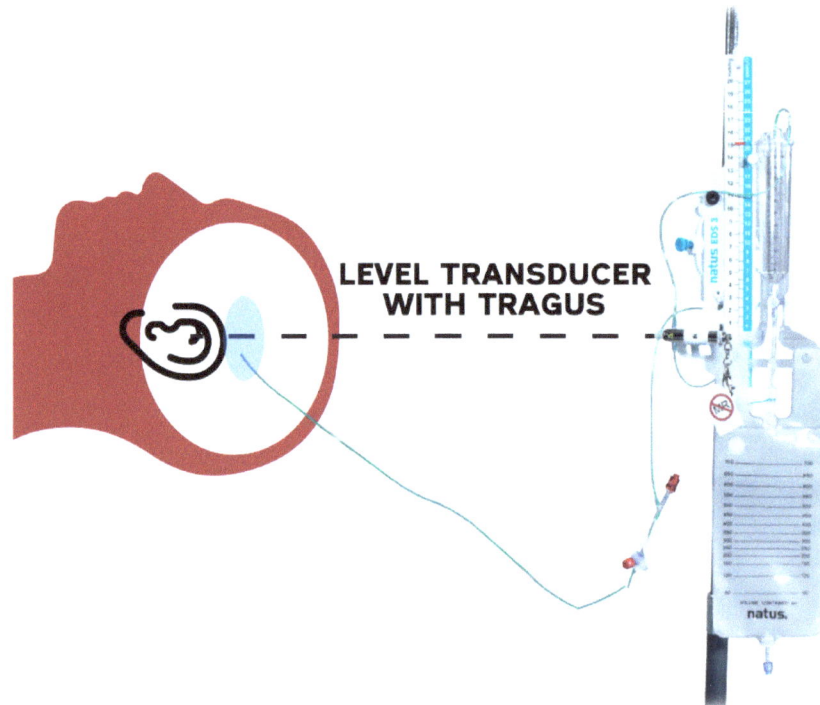

LEVEL TRANSDUCER WITH TRAGUS

Other Neuro ICU Monitoring Technology[9]
- **Optic Ultrasound: monitors ICP by measuring optic nerve diameter**
- **$SjVO_2$: fiberoptic catheters placed into IJ to measure cerebral oxygen supply, perfusion, and consumption**
- **$PbtiO_2$: brain tissue oxygenation monitoring, electrode placed on at-risk tissue**
- **Intracerebral Microdialysis: pulls minute amount of blood out to measure brain neurochemistry**

Treating Increased ICP
- Supportive care: A-B-C
- Elevate head of bed approximately 30°
- Treat seizures
- Provide sedation
- Neuro ICU:
  - Treat fever
  - Consider deep sedation: Barbiturates (careful dosing!)

Hyperventilation[6]
- May consider CONTROLLED/TARGETED hyperventilation if immediate signs of impending herniation
  - Increase minute volume 20%
  - Target $PaCO_2$ 28-30

DO NOT HYPERVENTILATE IN THE FIELD OR WITH A BVM

Hyperosmolar Therapy: Mannitol[6]
- Osmotic diuretic
- Must monitor serum osmolality
- May cause hypovolemia due to diuresis
- Crystallizes in the cold

Hypertonic Saline[6]
- Usually 3% saline
- Bolus 250 mL over 10-30 min
- Sodium goal: 150-155

Stroke

Ischemic Stroke[6]
- **Think FAST:**
  - **Facial weakness**
  - **Arm weakness**
  - **Speech difficulty**
  - **Time to call 911**
- **Cincinnati Stroke Scale**
  - **Facial droop**
  - **Pronator drift**
  - **Speech abnormality**
- **NIH Stroke Scale**
  - **EVERY stroke patient will be examined based on the NIH stroke scale in hospital**
    - **Baseline**
    - **Serial**
    - **Post-intervention**
    - **tPA typically not given below NIH 5 or above NIH 22**

Penumbra
- **Area surrounding the dead tissue is hypoxic, irritated, and is salvageable**
- **Act fast to save penumbra**

Stroke Treatment: Basics[6]
- **Supportive care**
- **$SpO_2 > 94\%$**
- **Check blood glucose**
- **Monitor EKG**

Ischemic Stroke: BP Management[6]
- **Permissive hypertension**
  - **Too much HTN causes cerebral edema**
- **BP goal is generally:**
  - **Systolic: 140-160**
  - **Diastolic: 70-90**
  - **<180/105 before, during, and 24hrs after tPA**
- **Hypotension**
  - **Can indicate herniation**
  - **Worsens outcomes if iatrogenic (sedatives, aggressive antihypertensive therapy)**

Thrombolytics: tPA vs. TNK[8]
- **Tissue Plasminogen Activator**
  - **0.9 mg/kg, maximum dose 90mg***
  - **10% dose bolus over 1 minute, 90% over 60-minute infusion**
  - **Many safety concerns and inclusion/exclusion criteria (e.g., hemorrhage)**
- **Tenecteplase**
  - **Cheaper**
  - **More favorable pharmacologic profile**
  - **Given in a single bolus**

Stroke dosing

Endovascular Therapy[6]
- **"Gold standard" in ischemic stroke care**
- **Clot retrieval in interventional radiology suite**
- **Indication is for LVO**
  - **Last known normal time: 16-24 hours**

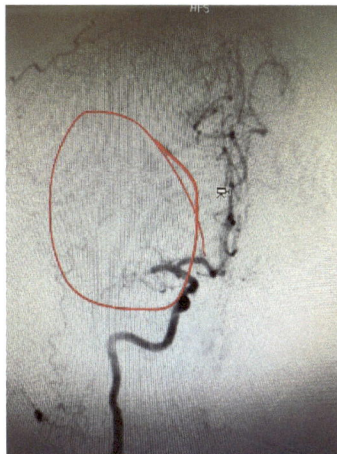

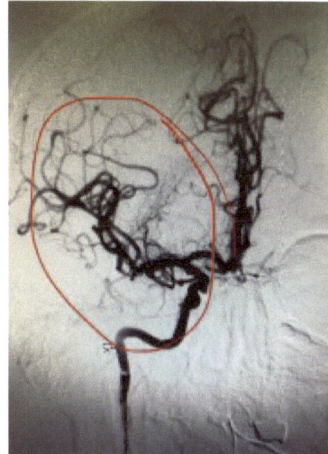

Decompressive Hemicrainectomy[6]
- **Goal: save the patient's life**
- **Candidates:**
  - **<60 YOA**
  - **>50% stroke volume**
  - **NIH score >16**
- **Must be done within 48 hours of onset**

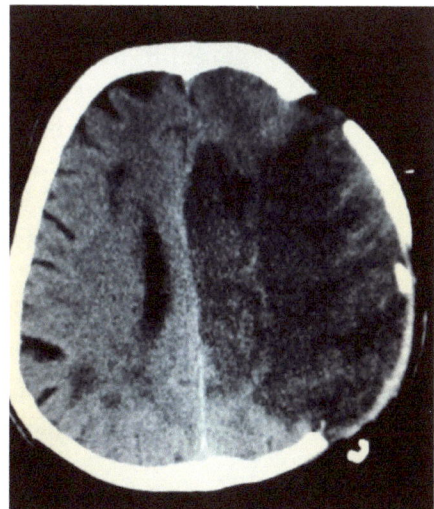

Hemorrhagic Stroke[1,6]

- **High mortality rate**
- **3% of strokes annually in USA**
- **Incidence doubles every 10 years after age 35**
- **High rate of associated problems**
    - **Cause is often cardiovascular related**
    - **Seizures in 16%**
    - **Hydrocephalus**
    - **Fever, infection**
- **Seizures should be treated**
- **Reversing anticoagulation is crucial**
    - **Vitamin K**
    - **K-Centra**
- **Blood pressure must be carefully controlled**
    - **Labetalol (beta blocker, push)**
    - **Nicardipine (calcium channel blocker, infusion)**
- **TREAT THE PATIENT'S PAIN**

Intraparenchymal Hemorrhage[6]

- **Results from hypertension**
- **Treat with antihypertensives**
- **BP Goal: ~140 mmHg systolic**

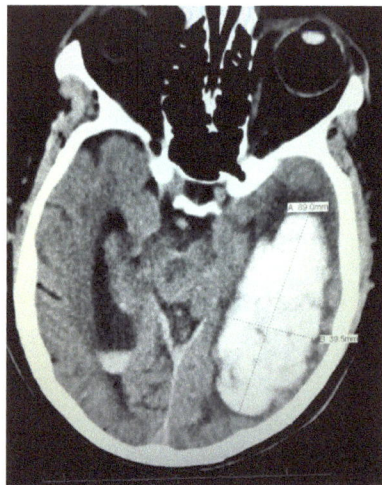

Subarachnoid Hemorrhage[1,6]

- **Acute onset**
    - **"Worst headache of life" and "thunderclap"**
    - **Treat hypertension**
        - **Target BP: <160 systolic, <110 diastolic**
    - **Many co-morbidities associated with SAH**
        - **Myocardial injury from catecholamine surge**
        - **Fever, infection**
        - **About 25% will have seizures**
        - **About 20% will have pulmonary complications**
        - **Hyperglycemia**
    - **Starfish sign on CT**

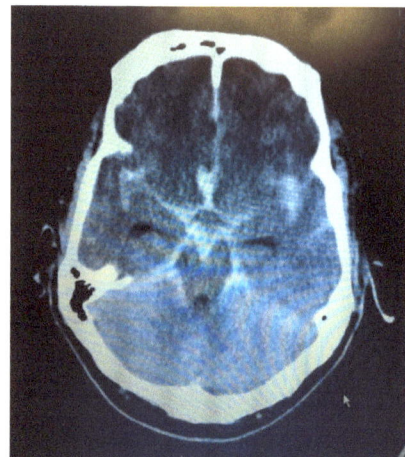

Neurologic Emergencies

Altered Mental Status[2]
AEIOU TIPS:
     Acidosis
     Epilepsy
     Insulin
     Overdose
     Uremia
     Trauma
     Infection
     Psychosis
     Seizures

Coma[2]
- **"Unarousable unresponsiveness"**
- **GLASGOW COMA SCALE (3-15)**
    - **Eye opening (1-4)**
    - **Verbal responsiveness (1-5)**
    - **Motor function (1-6)**

Delirium[2]
- **"Acute brain failure"**
- **Transient alteration of sensorium**
- **Often waxes and wanes**
- **Different from dementia**
    - **Fixed and irreversible brain changes**
    - **ICU Delirium**
    - **Interrupted circadian rhythm, constant provocation, pharmacotherapy side effects**

Seizures[10]
- PROVOKED: identified proximate cause
  - AEIOU-TIPS
- UNPROVOKED: no identified proximate cause
  - Epilepsy is a condition of recurrent unprovoked seizures
- Suspect unwitnessed seizure with:
  - Unexplained confusion or behavior change
  - Sudden falls with no recall or warning
  - Recurrent events occurring in various circumstances
  - Arousal from sleep with confusion

Status Epilepticus[6]
- Continuous clinical or EEG evidence of seizure for > 5 minutes
-OR-
- Recurrent seizure activity without a return to baseline between seizures
- Two types:
  - Convulsive
  - Non-convulsive: subtle and variable symptoms

Seizure Treatment[4,6]
- First line: Benzodiazepines
- Second line agents
  - Phenytoin (Dilantin) or Fosphenytoin
  - Valproic acid (Depakote)
  - Levetiracetam (Keppra)
  - Phenobarbital
  - Other agents (3rd and 4th line)
  - Propofol
  - Ketamine

Brain Tumors[5]
- Increased ICP
- Incidence: 30 per 100,000
- Headache most common symptom
- Focal seizures common
- Most primary brain tumors are idiopathic

Encephalopathy[6]
"Any diffuse disease of the brain that alters structure or function."
- Delirium is the most common presenting symptom
- Types
  - Acute: Toxic, metabolic, toxic-metabolic
  - Chronic: Slow and progressive alteration
  - Treat underlying pathology

Meningitis[3,6]

- Inflammation of the meninges
- Usually bacterial or viral
- Varied clinical presentation
  - Fever with headache
  - Signs of increased ICP: nausea, vomiting
  - New-onset seizures
  - Rash
  - Photophobia
  - Neck pain, neck stiffness
    - Brudzinski's Sign: Position patient supine and passively flex their neck, they will flex their hip and knee
    - Kernig's Sign: Severe hamstring stiffness, unable to straighten leg when the hip is flexed 90°

Neuromuscular Disorders[6]
- Guillain-Barré
  - Acute immune-mediated
  - Flaccid ascending weakness with areflexia
  - Severe cases: neuromuscular respiratory failure
- Myasthenia Gravis
  - Autoimmune disease affecting the post-synaptic junction
  - Ptosis is classic finding, extremity weakness, dyspnea
- Botulism
  - Spore-forming bacteria
  - Descending flaccid paralysis with intact mental status and no fever (classic triad)

questions:

1. The patient is a 43-year-old male with an acute onset of a "nuclear headache" along with photophobia and vomiting. His blood pressure is 204/138.
   - What condition do you suspect?
   - What CT findings would you expect to find?
   - Would you treat his BP? Agent? Target BP?

2. Where should the transducer be leveled in the patient with ICP monitoring?

   a. Foramen of Monro
   b. Foramen of Ovale
   c. Foramen Magnum
   d. Phlebostatic Axis

Chapter 12 citations:

1. AANN. (2018). Nursing Care of the Patient with Aneurysmal Subarachnoid Hemorrhage. Available: https://aann.org/uploads/Publications/CPGs/Nursing_Care_Patient_Aneurysmal_CPG_S AH_final2.pdf
2. Angela Cirilli. Brian Wiener. (15 May 2020). Evaluation and Treatment of Altered Mental Status in the Emergency Department. Emergency Medicine Reports. Available: https://www.reliasmedia.com/articles/146212-evaluation-and-treatment-of-altered-mental-status-in-the-emergency-department
3. Hersi K, Gonzalez FJ, Kondamudi NP. Meningitis. [Updated 2022 Aug 14]. In: StatPearls [Internet]. Treasure Island (FL): StatPearls Publishing; 2022 Jan-. Available from: https://www.ncbi.nlm.nih.gov/books/NBK459360/
4. Howing CE, Razi F, Hakmeh W. Resolution of status epilepticus after ketamine administration. Am J Emerg Med. 2022 Apr;54:328.e1-328.e2. doi: 10.1016/j.ajem.2021.10.052. Epub 2021 Nov 3. PMID: 34763960.
5. Eric Wong. Julian Wu. (2022). Overview of the Clinical Features and Diagnosis of Brain Tumors in Adults. Up-to-Date.
6. Jack Jallo. Jacqueline Urtecho. (2021). The Jefferson Manual for Neurocritical Care.
7. Nag K, Singh DR, Shetti AN, Kumar H, Sivashanmugam T, Parthasarathy S. Sugammadex: A revolutionary drug in neuromuscular pharmacology. Anesth Essays Res. 2013 Sep-Dec;7(3):302-6. doi: 10.4103/0259-1162.123211. PMID: 25885973; PMCID: PMC4173552.
8. Salim Rezaie, "Tenecteplase vs Alteplase in Acute Ischemic Stroke", REBEL EM blog, June 16, 2022. Available at: https://rebelem.com/tenecteplase-vs-alteplase-in-acute-ischemic-stroke/.
9. Shane Musick. Anthony Alberico. (2021). Neurologic Assessment of the Neurocritical Care Patient. Frontiers in Neurology: 22 March 2021. doi: 10.3389/fneur.2021.588989
10. Tina Shih. (2022). Seizure and Epilepsy in Older Adults: Etiology, Clinical Presentation, and Diagnosis. Up-to-Date.

Chapter 13: Trauma & burns

General trauma principles

Trauma Scoring[3]
- **Injury Severity Scale (score: 1-75)**
- **Adjusted ISS**
    - **1: Minor**
    - **2: Moderate**
    - **3: Serious**
    - **4: Severe**
    - **5: Critical**
    - **6: Maximum**

Kinematics of Trauma[3]
- **An object in motion stays in motion…**
- **Force = Mass x Acceleration**
- **Momentum = mass x velocity**
- **Axis of impact:**
    - **Forward: well tolerated**
    - **Vertical: moderately tolerated**
    - **Lateral: poorly tolerated**

Deceleration and Shearing Forces[3]
- **MVA: Frontal Impact**
    - **Down and Under Pathway**
        - **Occurs early in the crash sequence**
        - **Lower extremity and abdominal trauma**
    - **Up and Over**
        - **Chest hits steering wheel (shearing forces)**
        - **Head hits windshield (axial loading)**
- **MVA: Lateral Impacts[3]**
    - **Can be devastating due to lateral forces on body**
    - **Shearing forces**
- **MVA: Rear Impact[3]**
    - **High likelihood for c-spine injury**
- **Rollovers**
    - **Unpredictable injury patterns**
    - **Low mortality with seatbelt use**

Falls[3]

- **Kinetic energy is related to height**
- **Type of surface**
- **Which body part struck the ground first?**

Penetrating Trauma: Cavitation[3]

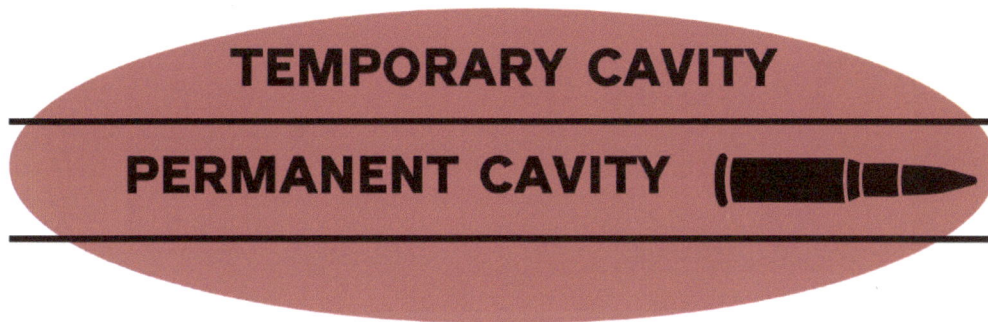

TEMPORARY CAVITY

PERMANENT CAVITY

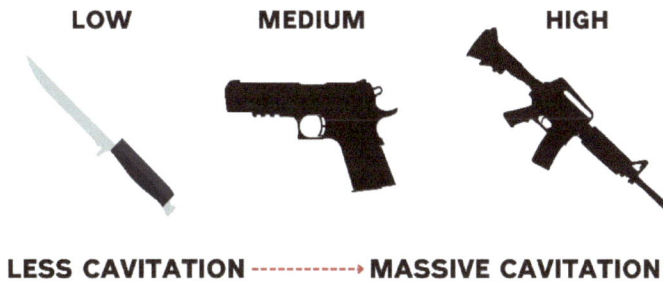

LOW   MEDIUM   HIGH

LESS CAVITATION ----------> MASSIVE CAVITATION

Cavitation & Fragmenting

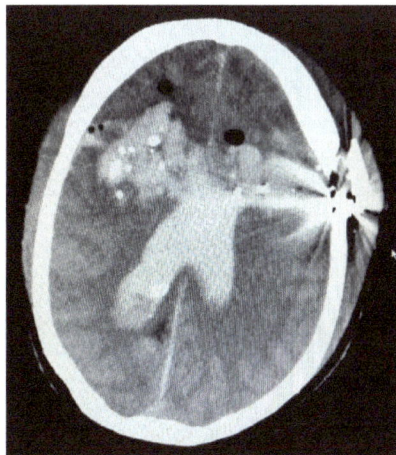

Traumatic Shock[3]

- **Hemorrhagic shock**

- **Inflammation**
- **Toxin release**
- **Coagulopathies**

Shock Index

HEART RATE
÷
SYSTOLIC BP

Normal: <0.7
Shock: >0.9
Poor outcomes: >1.3

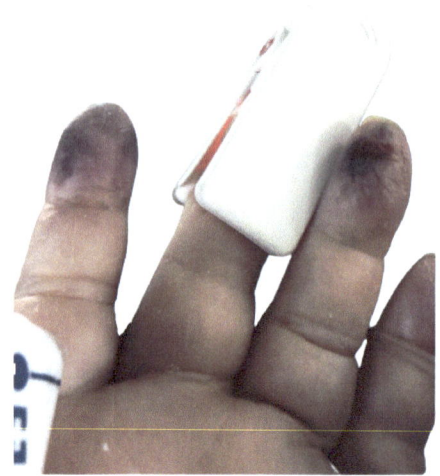

Critical Shock:
- **SBP <100**
- **HR >100**
- **HCT <32%**
- **pH <7.25**

Stop the Bleeding[2]
- **EARLY TOURNIQUET APPLICATION**
- **Direct pressure**
- **Elevation**
- **Pressure point**

Thromboelastography (TEG)[15]

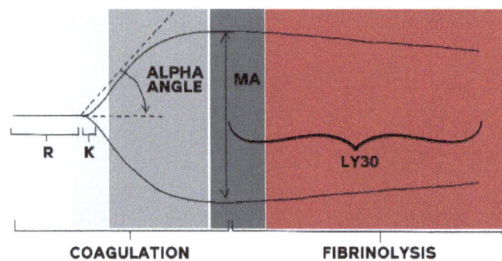

COMPONENTS	DEFINITION	NORMAL VALUES	PROBLEM WITH?	TREATMENT
R Time	Time to start forming clot	5 - 10 minutes	Coagulation Factors	FFP
K Time	Time until clot reaches a fixed strength	1 - 3 minutes	Fibrinogen	Cryoprecipitate
Alpha angle	Speed of fibrin accumulation	53 -72 degrees	Fibrinogen	Cryoprecipitate
Maximum Amplitude (MA)	Highest vertical amplitude of the TEG	50 - 70 mm	Platelets	Platelets and/or DDAVP
Lysis at 30 minutes (LY30)	Percentage of amplitude reduction 30 minutes after maximum amplitude	0 - 8 %	Excess Fibrinolysis	Tranexemic Acid and/or Aminocaproic Acid

Disseminated Intravascular Coagulation[7]

- **Coagulopathy in concert with microvascular thrombosis**
- **Thrombocytopenia, abnormal coags**
- **Elevated D-dimer**
- **Continuous bleeding**

The Lethal Triad[3]

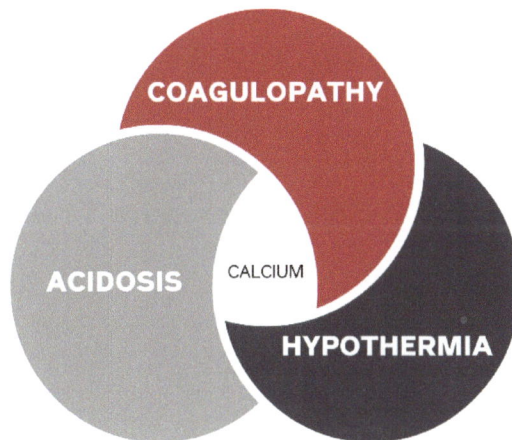

Hypothermia[3]
- **Heating fluids**
- **Heated blankets**
- **Cabin temperature**

Calcium[14, 16]
- **The Lethal Triad is now the "Lethal Diamond"**
- **Calcium is critical for clotting**
- **Ionized Calcium: "free calcium"**
- **Calcium is bound up by citrate in PRBC administration**

TXA[2, 14, 17]
- **Major trauma causes hyperfibrinolysis**
- **Prevents plasmin from stabilizing the fibrin matrix**
- **Must be given within 3 hours of injury**
  - **IV**
  - **TXA-soaked gauze**
  - **Nebulized**

Isotonic Crystalloid[14]
- 0.9% NSS (pH 5.5)
- Lactated Ringer's (pH 6.5)
- NEITHER should be 1st line for traumatic shock

Blood Products[5,14]
- PRBC
  - Increases oxygen carrying capacity
- Plasma
  - Give if there is any clotting deficiency
- Platelets
  - "Clump" together to form clots

Low Titer O Whole Blood[5,14,18]
- The BEST blood product to provide in hemorrhagic shock
- There is no universal definition of "low titer"
- Reduces the amount of citrate delivered to the patient
- Downside: short shelf life, expensive

Damage Control Resuscitation[5, 14]
- GOAL: MINIMIZE SHOCK BURDEN
  - Restore homeostasis
  - Prevent hypoxia
  - Reduce oxygen debt
  - Mitigate Coagulopathy
- Use Low Titer O Whole Blood (LTOWB) or 1:1:1 Ratio of PRBC:Plasma:Plt

Permissive Hypotension[14]
- Goal: perfuse vital organs without disrupting clot formation or expediting exsanguination
- Over-resuscitation is harmful
  - Increases hemorrhage
  - Destroys established clots
- SBP minimum goal: 90-100 mmHg
  - 110 mmHg if associated CNS involvement

DOES NOT APPLY TO ISOLATED HEAD TRAUMA

Transfusion Reactions[12]
- **Hemolytic**
  - **Fever, chills, flank pain**
- **Febrile**
  - **Non-hemolytic**
  - **Managed with acetaminophen**
- **TACO**
  - **Circulatory overload**
- **TRALI**
  - **Acute lung injury, similar to ARDS**

Head-to-toe trauma

Facial Trauma: LeFort Fractures[3]

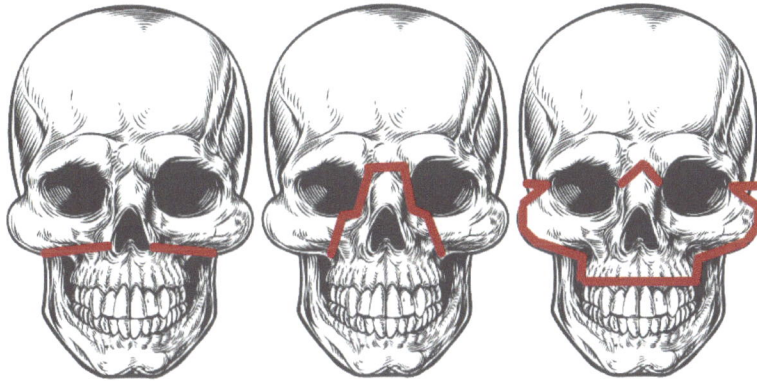

Eye Trauma[3]
- **Often concomitant with head trauma**
- **Instruct patient to not strain or squeeze eyelids shut**
- **Post traumatic floaters and a visual field defect suggest a retinal detachment**
- **Ocular compartment syndrome is managed with a lateral canthotomy**

Extremity Trauma[3]
- **Re-align if possible**
- **Femur may conceal large amounts of bleeding**
- **Signs of vascular injury**
  - **Active or pulsatile hemorrhage**
  - **Clinical signs of limb ischemia**
  - **Pulsatile or expanding hematoma**
  - **Diminished or absent pulses**
  - **Bruit or thrill suggesting AV fistula**

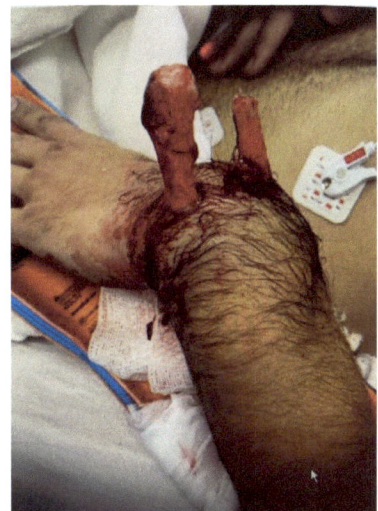

Compartment Syndrome[3]
6 P's:
- Pain
- Paresthesia
- Poikilothermia
- Pallor
- Paralysis
- Pulselessness

POCUS: eFAST Exam[11]
- RUQ
- Pelvis
- LUQ
- Cardiac
- Lungs

Chest Trauma

Aortic Injury[8, 9]
- High mortality
- Shearing forces, lateral impact
- Often presents with hypotension and AMS
- Shearing forces causes tearing of the aorta
  - Causes tearing, flapping, and pseudoaneurysm
- Chest X-ray
  - Widened mediastinum
  - Enlarged aortic knob
  - Large left-hemothorax
  - Trachea may deviate rightward
- Treatment
  - Anti-impulse therapy
  - Heart rate is top priority
  - SBP goal: less than 100 mmHg
    - Beta blockers are first-line
    - Esmolol is ideal first-agent
- Rib Fractures[3]

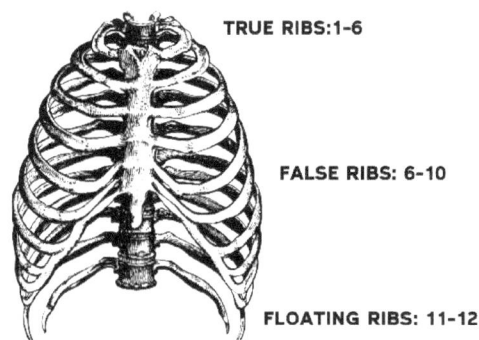

TRUE RIBS:1-6

FALSE RIBS: 6-10

FLOATING RIBS: 11-12

Pneumothorax[2,3]

- Size matters: 14 gauge, 3.25"
- Sites
    - Anterior: 2nd ICS midclavicular
    - Axillary: 5th ICS anterior axillary
- SpO_2 goal: >90%
- Needle Thoracostomy

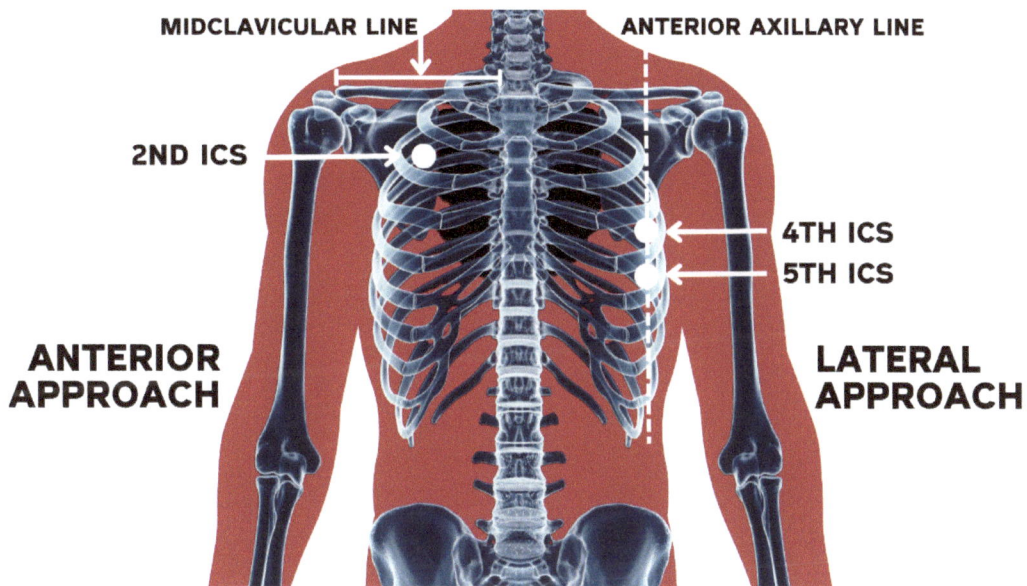

MIDCLAVICULAR LINE   ANTERIOR AXILLARY LINE

2ND ICS   4TH ICS   5TH ICS

ANTERIOR APPROACH   LATERAL APPROACH

Hemothorax[3]
- Should be drained
- Can resuscitate with autotransfusion
- Retained hemothorax is harmful

Pulmonary Contusion[3]
- Highly associated with MVA
- Respiratory distress that appears over time
- Supportive treatment
- Avoid over fluid resuscitation
- Encourage coughing, deep breathing
- Supplemental oxygen PRN

Penetrating Cardiac Injury[3]
- 52% stabbings
- 42% GSW
- Ventricles are at greatest risk for injury because of positioning
- Majority of injuries are simple lacerations

Pericardial Tamponade[2]
- **Fluid accumulation in pericardial sack**
- **Causes obstructive shock**
  - **Heart cannot fill nor contract**
- **EKG: electrical alternans**
- **Beck's Triad**

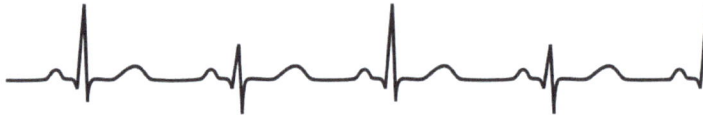

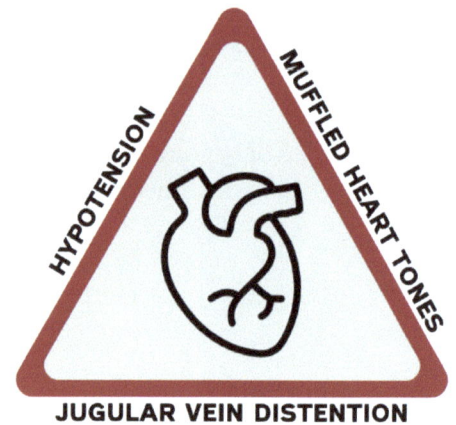

- **Treatment:**
  - **Pericardiocentesis**
  - **Fluid bolus (temporizing measure)**
  - **Pericardial window**

Blunt Cardiac Injury[3]
- **Presents with:**
  - **Tamponade**
  - **Hemorrhage**
  - **Severe cardiac dysfunction**
- **May cause:**
  - **Septal rupture and valvular dysfunction**
  - **Delayed heart failure without initial symptoms**

Tracheobronchial Injury[3]
- **Subcutaneous air may be observed**
- **Classic presentation:**
  - **Pneumothorax not responsive to evacuation**
  - **Air leakage through chest tube**
  - **Persistent recurrent pneumothorax**
- **Extreme care when intubating**
  - **Insert deep right mainstem**

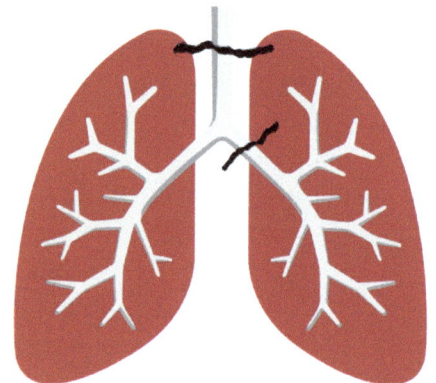

Diaphragmatic Hernia[3]
- **Usually on left side**
- **Most commonly from penetrating trauma**
- **Symptoms vary from none to critical**

Abdominal trauma

Liver Injury[3]
- Commonly injured due to size
- Extremely vascular
- Different grades of liver injury

Splenic Trauma[3]
- Commonly injured
- Causes referred shoulder pain
  - Kehr's sign
- Have high index of suspicion
- Children quite susceptible
- Can hold large amount of blood

Bowel and Stomach[3]
- Most common injury due to seat belts
- Low risk of peritonitis if stomach ruptures
- High risk of peritonitis if bowel ruptures

Pelvic Trauma[3,13]
- Highly vascular
- High potential for shock
- Mortality up to 40%
- POCUS is ineffective
- Perform stabilization in presence of mechanism for pelvic fracture and signs of shock

REBOA[1,8,9,14]
- Occludes aorta
  - Zone 1: thoracic trauma
  - Zone 2: abdominal trauma
  - Zone 3: pelvic trauma
- Not for thoracic *aortic* injury
- Success in combat environments, post-partum hemorrhage

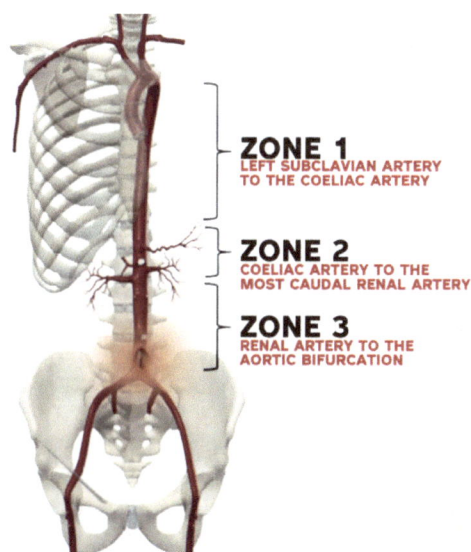

ZONE 1
LEFT SUBCLAVIAN ARTERY TO THE COELIAC ARTERY

ZONE 2
COELIAC ARTERY TO THE MOST CAUDAL RENAL ARTERY

ZONE 3
RENAL ARTERY TO THE AORTIC BIFURCATION

Genitourinary Trauma[3]
- 10% of abdominal trauma patients will have concomitant GU injury
- 90% of injuries are renal injuries from blunt trauma
- Hematuria is an important finding but may be absent in up to 45% of cases
- Magnitude of hematuria does not correlate with degree of injury

Special Situations

Pediatric Trauma[6]
- **Head trauma common due to proportionally large heads**
- **Less thoracic protection**
- **Less abdominal protection**
- **Delayed signs of shock**
    - **MINIMUM SBP: 70 + (2 x age in years)**

Trauma in Pregnancy[3]
- **MVA most common major trauma**
- **Placental abruption most common injury**
- **Maternal shock = 80% fetal mortality rate**
- **Supine hypotensive syndrome**
    - **Weight of gravid uterus on IVC**
- **Aggressive resuscitation**
- **Target SpO_2 >95%**

Crush Injuries[3,4]
- **Entrapment >24 hours: high mortality**
- **Tourniquets are not recommended**
- **Crush Syndrome: organ dysfunction (AKI)**
    - **Myoglobinemia**
    - **Rhabdomyolysis**
    - **Hyperkalemia**

Traumatic Asphyxia[3]
- **Due to significant increase in thoracic pressure**
- **Often not fatal**
- **Classic presentation:**
    - **Cervicofacial cyanosis**
    - **Subconjunctival hemorrhage**
    - **Petechia on face, neck, and chest**

Blast Injuries[3]

1: PRIMARY
pressure injury

2: SECONDARY
shrapnel

3: TERTIARY
acceleration, deceleration

4: QUATERNARY
thermal injury

5: QUINARY
chemical, biologic, radiologic, nuclear effects

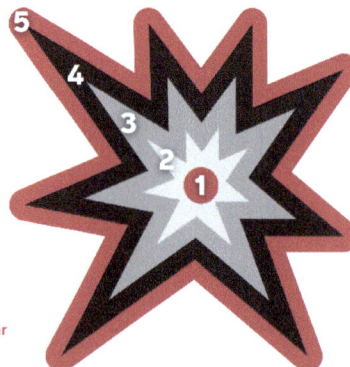

QUESTIONS:

1. You are transferring a trauma patient from a community hospital to a level 1 trauma center. She presented with back pain after a high-speed MVA. CXR shows a widened mediastinum. Which of the following symptoms is the first issue that should be managed?

   a. BP 90/40
   b. HR 93
   c. RR 30
   d. Hgb 7.4

2. A 5-year-old was run over by a stagecoach. What is the minimum systolic blood pressure for this patient?

   a. 80 mmHg
   b. 90 mmHg
   c. 60 mmHg
   d. 72 mmHg

Chapter 13: trauma citations:

1. Castellini G, Gianola S, Biffi A, Porcu G, Fabbri A, Ruggieri MP, Coniglio C, Napoletano A, Coclite D, D'Angelo D, Fauci AJ, Iacorossi L, Latina R, Salomone K, Gupta S, Iannone P, Chiara O; Italian National Institute of Health guideline working group on Major Trauma. Resuscitative endovascular balloon occlusion of the aorta (REBOA) in patients with major trauma and uncontrolled haemorrhagic shock: a systematic review with meta-analysis. World J Emerg Surg. 2021 Aug 12;16(1):41. doi: 10.1186/s13017-021-00386-9. PMID: 34384452; PMCID: PMC8358549.
2. Committee on TCCC. (2021). Tactical Combat Casualty Care Guidelines for Medical Personnel. Available: https://deployedmedicine.com/content/475
3. Feliciano, Mattox, and Moore. (2021). Trauma 9th Ed. McGraw Hill.
4. Godat, L., Doucet, J. (2022). Severe Crush Injury in Adults. Up-to-Date.
5. Kutcher, Matthew. Cohen, Mitchell. (2022). Coagulopathy in Trauma Patients. Up-To-Date.
6. Lee, Lois. Farrell, Caitlin. (2022). Trauma Management: Unique Pediatric Considerations. Up-to-Date.
7. Leung, Lawrence. (2022). Evaluation and management of disseminated intravascular coagulation (DIC) in adults. Up-to-Date.
8. Nechis. (2022). Management of Blunt Thoracic Aortic Injury. Up-to-Date.
9. Neschis, Vignon, Lang. (2022). Clinical features and diagnosis of blunt thoracic aortic injury. Up-to-Date.
10. Paz MS, Mendez MD. Waddell Triad. 2022 Jul 18. In: StatPearls [Internet]. Treasure Island (FL): StatPearls Publishing; 2022 Jan–. PMID: 30725779.
11. Stringham, Dustin. Hart, Kasey. (2020). POCUS: The Inside View.
12. Tobian, Aaron. (2022). Approach to the Patient with a Suspected Acute Transfusion Reaction. Up-to-Date.
13. Tullington JE, Blecker N. Pelvic Trauma. [Updated 2022 May 8]. In: StatPearls [Internet]. Treasure Island (FL): StatPearls Publishing; 2022 Jan-. Available from: https://www.ncbi.nlm.nih.gov/books/NBK556070/
14. United States Army. (2019). Damage Control Resuscitation Clinical Practice Guideline.
15. Brill JB, Brenner M, Duchesne J, Roberts D, Ferrada P, Horer T, Kauvar D, Khan M, Kirkpatrick A, Ordonez C, Perreira B, Priouzram A, Cotton BA. The Role of TEG and ROTEM in Damage Control Resuscitation. Shock. 2021 Dec 1;56(1S):52-61. doi: 10.1097/SHK.0000000000001686. PMID: 33769424; PMCID: PMC8601668.
16. Wray JP, Bridwell RE, Schauer SG, Shackelford SA, Bebarta VS, Wright FL, Bynum J, Long B. The diamond of death: Hypocalcemia in trauma and resuscitation. Am J Emerg Med. 2021 Mar;41:104-109. doi: 10.1016/j.ajem.2020.12.065. Epub 2020 Dec 28. PMID: 33421674.
17. Roberts I, Shakur H, Coats T, Hunt B, Balogun E, Barnetson L, Cook L, Kawahara T, Perel P, Prieto-Merino D, Ramos M, Cairns J, Guerriero C. The CRASH-2 trial: a randomised controlled trial and economic evaluation of the effects of tranexamic acid on death, vascular occlusive events and transfusion requirement in bleeding trauma patients. Health Technol Assess. 2013 Mar;17(10):1-79. doi: 10.3310/hta17100. PMID: 23477634; PMCID: PMC4780956.

18. 10/17/2018 <u>Christa A. L. Arefieva, MS, MSIV</u> , <u>Bryan Chen, MD</u> , <u>Theodore T. Redman, MD, MPH</u> , <u>Andrew D. Fisher, MPAS, PA-C, LP</u>; Available https://www.emra.org/emresident/article/group-o-whole-blood/

NEUROTRAUMA

Monro-Kellie Doctrine:
There is a fixed, finite volume within the cranial vault; if one component increases, another must decrease

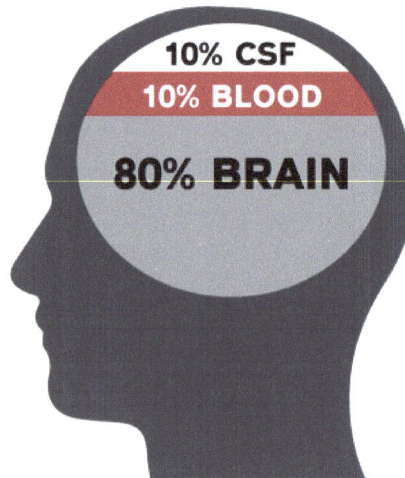

Increased ICP: Cushing's Triad

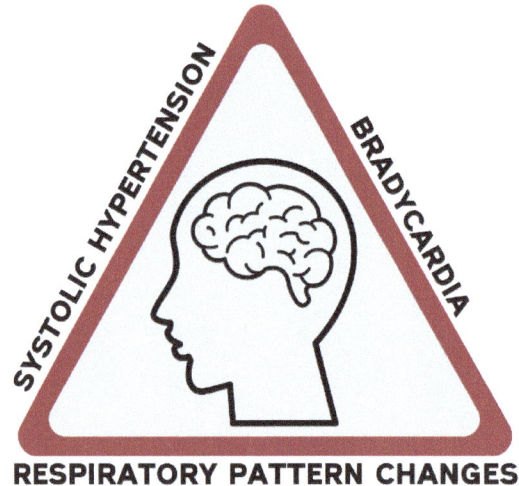

Pupils[1]
- Herniation may cause a dilated pupil.
- Damage to midbrain or compression of CN III may occur as the brain tissue herniates into the tentorial notch.
- Direct orbital trauma may also cause dilation and fixation in a "sizeable minority of cases."

Glasgow Coma Score

EYE OPENING

4 SPONTANEOUS

3 TO SOUND

2 TO PRESSURE

1 NONE

SPEECH

5 ORIENTED

4 CONFUSED

3 WORDS

2 SOUNDS

1 NONE

MOTOR FUNCTION

6 OBEYS COMMANDS

5 LOCALIZING

4 NORMAL FLEXION

3 ABNORMAL FLEXION

2 EXTENSION

1 NONE

Primary Neuro Injury[1,5]
- Forces of impact
- Primary insult

Secondary Neuro Injury[1,5]
- Hypoxia
- Ischemia
- Seizures
- Fever
- Hypoglycemia
- Excitotoxicity

Secondary Injury Killers in TBI[1,5]

HYPOTENSION

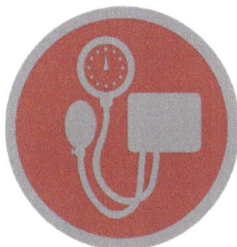

HYPOXIA

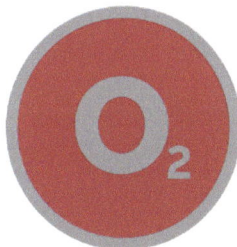

HYPERCARBIA

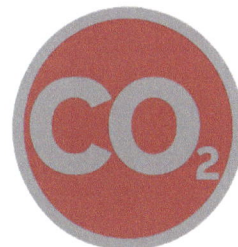

167

Skull Fractures[1,4]
- Linear: most common, low risk for acute neuro effects or long-term deficits
- Diastatic: involves cranial sutures
- Depressed: risk for pneumocephalus and infection

Basilar Skull Fracture[1]
- Postauricular or periorbital ecchymosis
- CSF leak from nose and/or ears
- Hemotympanum
- Risk of meningitis

TRAUMA INSIDE THE SKULL

Subarachnoid[1]
- Venous tears
- "Starfish" pattern on CT

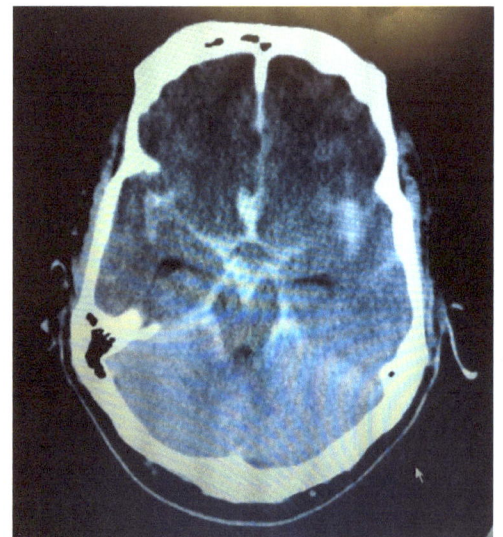

Subdural Hematoma[1]
- Slow, venous bleed
- "Venous lakes" pattern
- Result from higher magnitude forces
- Increased risk with brain atrophy
    - Alcoholics
    - Elderly

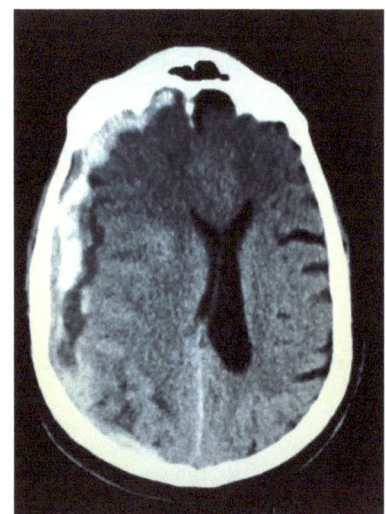

Epidural Bleeds[1,5]
- Middle meningeal artery
- Classic presentation:
    - **Head blow with LOC**
    - **Regains consciousness**
    - **Progressive decline in mental status**
- Lenticular shape

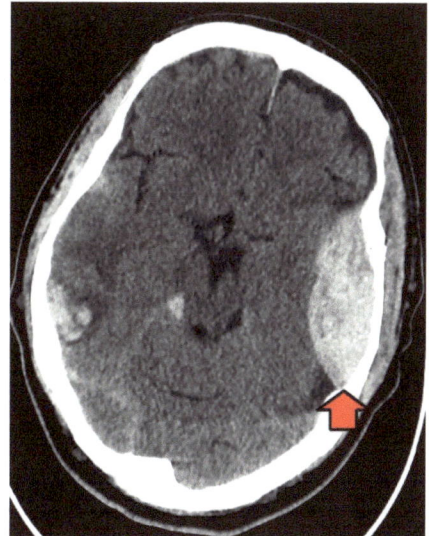

Diffuse Axonal Injury (DAI)[1,5]
- **Axons transected from rotation and shearing**
- **Typical presentation:**
    - **Coma or profound AMS**
    - **Initial: Normal head CT**
    - **Later: Punctate hemorrhages on CT**
- **Poor outcomes**

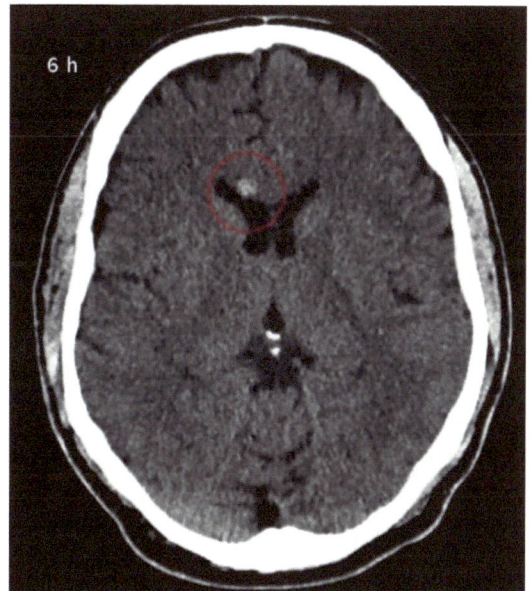

Concussion[1]
- **Does NOT require LOC**
- **Confusion**
- **Amnesia**
- **Nausea and vomiting**
- **Difficulty concentrating**
- **Vertigo**
- **Insomnia**
- **Abnormal coordination**

TBI Treatment Guidelines[1,3]

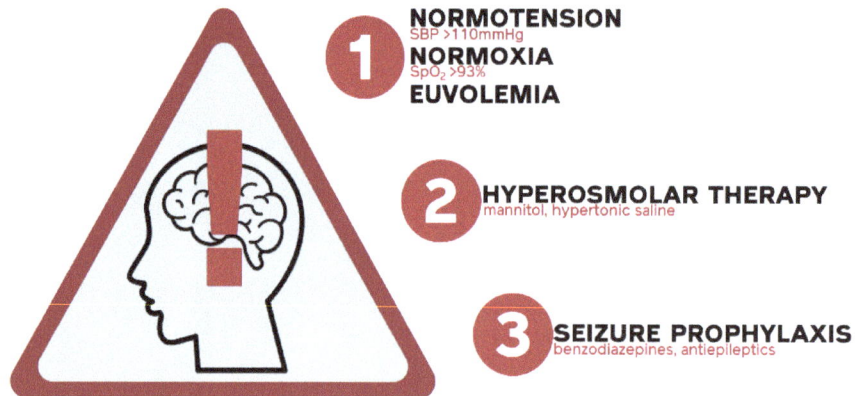

1. **NORMOTENSION**
   SBP >110mmHg
   NORMOXIA
   SpO2 >93%
   EUVOLEMIA

2. **HYPEROSMOLAR THERAPY**
   mannitol, hypertonic saline

3. **SEIZURE PROPHYLAXIS**
   benzodiazepines, antiepileptics

Other TBI Treatment Info[1,3]
- **Consider TXA**
- **Normal saline is preferred over Ringer's Lactate**

Spinal cord injuries

Common SCI Findings[2]:
- **Absent reflexes**
- **Bradycardia**
- **Reduced sensation**
- **Reduced muscle tone**
- **Urinary retention**
- **Priapism**

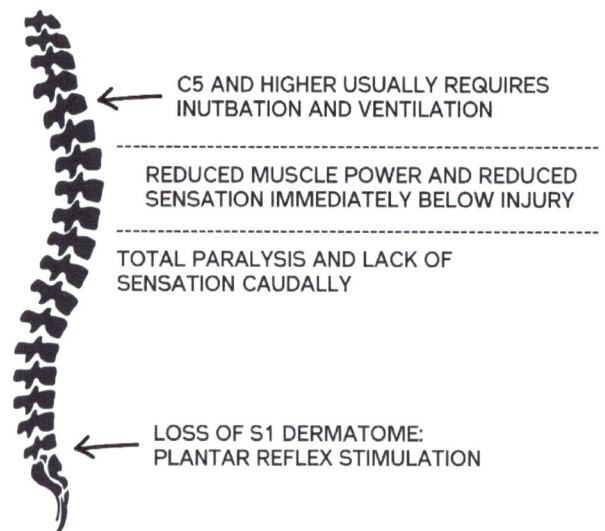

C5 AND HIGHER USUALLY REQUIRES INUTBATION AND VENTILATION

REDUCED MUSCLE POWER AND REDUCED SENSATION IMMEDIATELY BELOW INJURY

TOTAL PARALYSIS AND LACK OF SENSATION CAUDALLY

LOSS OF S1 DERMATOME: PLANTAR REFLEX STIMULATION

Neurogenic Shock[1]
- **Hypotension**
- **Bradycardia**
- **Skin changes below injury**

Spinal Shock[2]
- **Temporary motor dysfunction**
- **Possibly also bradycardia and/or hypotension**

Incomplete SCI

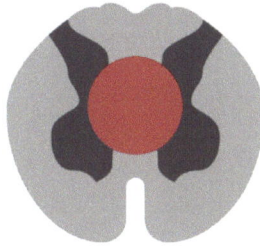

ANTERIOR CORD **CENTRAL CORD** **BROWN-SEQUARD**

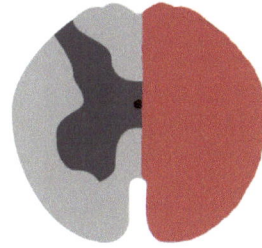

Anterior Cord Syndrome[1]

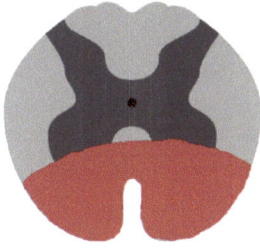

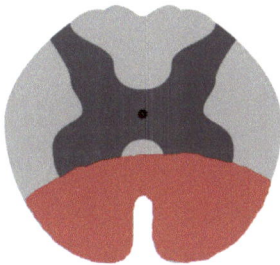

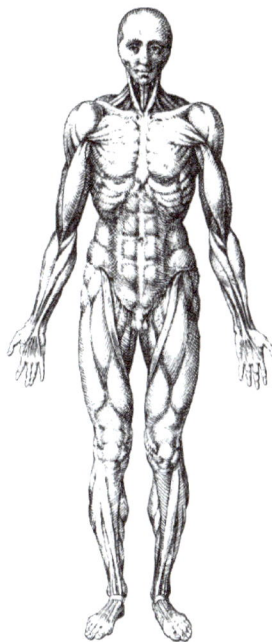

MOTOR DYSFUNCTION

PRESERVATION OF PRESSURE SENSATION

RETAINED PROPRIOCEPTION

Central Cord Syndrome[1]

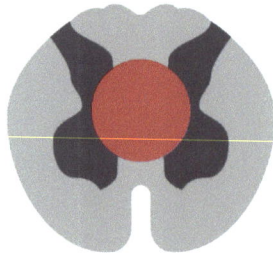

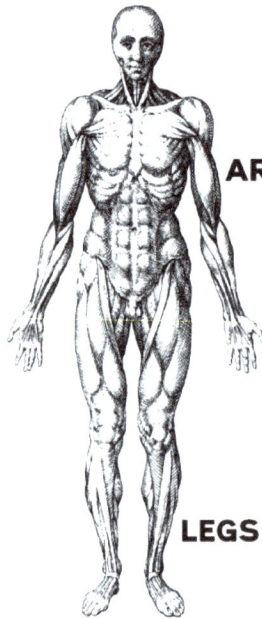

ARM WEAKNESS

"BURNING" HANDS

LEGS LESS WEAK THAN ARMS

Brown Sequard Syndrome[1]

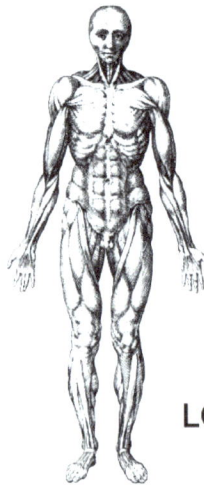

CONTRALATERAL
LOSS OF PAIN
LOSS OF HOT/COLD SENSATION

IPSILATERAL
LOSS OF MOTOR FUNCTION
LOSS OF PROPRIOCEPTION
LOSS OF LIGHT TOUCH SENSATION

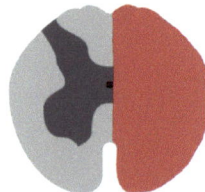

NEXUS Criteria
LOW probability of c-spine injury if:

- **No midline tenderness**
- **No focal neurologic deficit**
- **Normal alertness**
- **No intoxication**
- **No painful or distracting injury**

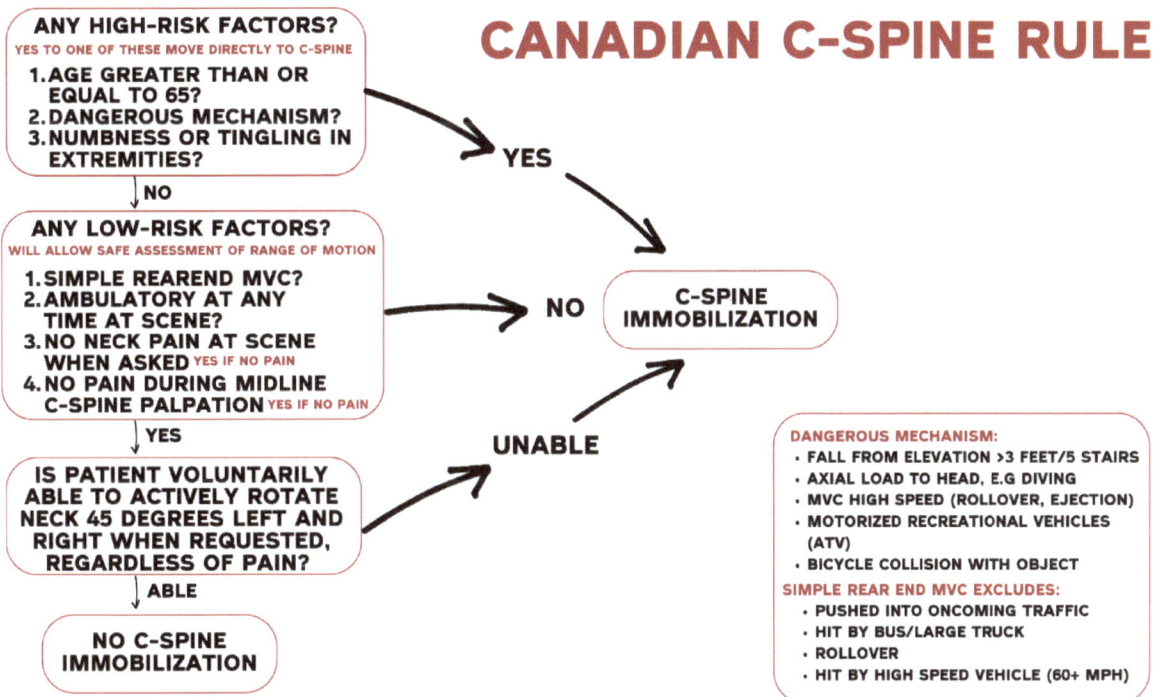

CANADIAN C-SPINE RULE

ANY HIGH-RISK FACTORS?
YES TO ONE OF THESE MOVE DIRECTLY TO C-SPINE
1. AGE GREATER THAN OR EQUAL TO 65?
2. DANGEROUS MECHANISM?
3. NUMBNESS OR TINGLING IN EXTREMITIES?

↓ NO

ANY LOW-RISK FACTORS?
WILL ALLOW SAFE ASSESSMENT OF RANGE OF MOTION
1. SIMPLE REAREND MVC?
2. AMBULATORY AT ANY TIME AT SCENE?
3. NO NECK PAIN AT SCENE WHEN ASKED YES IF NO PAIN
4. NO PAIN DURING MIDLINE C-SPINE PALPATION YES IF NO PAIN

↓ YES

IS PATIENT VOLUNTARILY ABLE TO ACTIVELY ROTATE NECK 45 DEGREES LEFT AND RIGHT WHEN REQUESTED, REGARDLESS OF PAIN?

↓ ABLE

NO C-SPINE IMMOBILIZATION

YES →

NO →

UNABLE →

C-SPINE IMMOBILIZATION

DANGEROUS MECHANISM:
- FALL FROM ELEVATION >3 FEET/5 STAIRS
- AXIAL LOAD TO HEAD, E.G DIVING
- MVC HIGH SPEED (ROLLOVER, EJECTION)
- MOTORIZED RECREATIONAL VEHICLES (ATV)
- BICYCLE COLLISION WITH OBJECT

SIMPLE REAR END MVC EXCLUDES:
- PUSHED INTO ONCOMING TRAFFIC
- HIT BY BUS/LARGE TRUCK
- ROLLOVER
- HIT BY HIGH SPEED VEHICLE (60+ MPH)

C-Collars: "BeCaUsE wE'Ve ALwaYs dOnE iT tHiS wAy."

TIME FOR A PARADIGM SHIFT?

LACK OF HIGH-QUALITY STUDIES SUPPORTING EFFICACY (PMID 32426850)

AN ALERT PATIENT WITH A NECK INJURY WILL DEMONSTRATE A SELF-PROTECTION MECHANISM, ENSURING INJURIES ARE NOT WORSENED. EVIDENCE IS NOW BUILDING THE SELF-EXTRICATION IN ALERT PATIENTS WITH MINIMAL OR NO C-SPINE IMMOBILIZATION IS SAFE (PMID 27748690)

MAY EXACERBATE C-SPINE INJURY. MAY INCREASE ICP BY AN AVERAGE OF 4.5 MMHG THROUGH JUGULAR VENOUS COMPRESSION (PMID 23962031)

KNOWN CORRELATION BETWEEN COLLAR USAGE AND ADVERSE EVENTS SUCH AS PRESSURE ULCERS, INFECTIONS, EXACERBATED SPINAL INJURY, AND HIGHER MORBIDITY (PMID 34537462)

questions:

3. Your patient was shot once in the chest. He is unable to move his right side. He can move his left side and does not feel anything when a 14-gauge catheter is inserted into his right wrist. You suspect:

   a. Brown-Sequard Syndrome
   b. Anterior Cord Syndrome
   c. Central Cord Syndrome
   d. Spinal Shock

4. Your patient is a 74-year-old alcoholic. Family called after noting new-onset confusion. While taking a history they tell you that the patient has had multiple falls over the last few days due to "being too drunk to walk." Which type of TBI would you suspect this patient may have?

   a. Central tentorial herniation
   b. Pontine hemorrhage
   c. Epidural hematoma
   d. Subdural hematoma

Chapter 13: Neurotrauma CITATIONS:

1. Feliciano, David V.; Feliciano, David V.; Mattox, Kenneth L.; Mattox, Kenneth L.; Moore, Ernest E.; Moore, Ernest E.. Trauma, Ninth Edition (p. 470). McGraw Hill LLC. Kindle Edition.
2. Hansebout, Robert. Kachur, Edward. (2022). Acute Traumatic Spinal Cord Injury. Up-to-Date.
3. Rajajee, Venkatakrishna. (2022). Management of acute moderate and severe traumatic brain injury. Up-to-Date.
4. Heegaard, William. (2022). Skull fractures in adults. Up-to-Date.
5. Williamson, Craig. Rajajee, Venkatakrishna. (2022). Traumatic Brain Injury: Epidemiology, Classification, and Pathophysiology. Up-to-Date.

Burns

Initial Assessment and Management[1]
- **Stop the burning process**
- **Remove clothing**
- **Maintain warmth**

Burn Zones

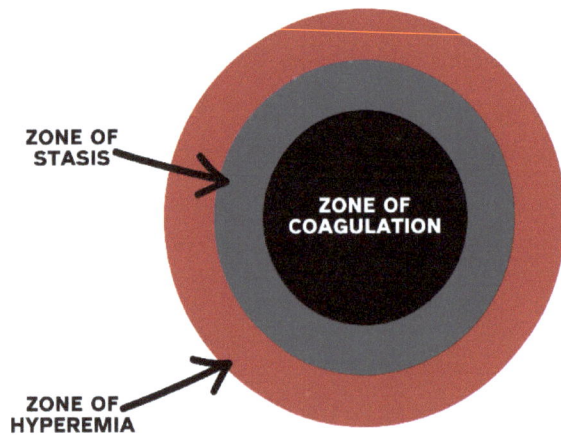

Grading Burn Injuries[1]

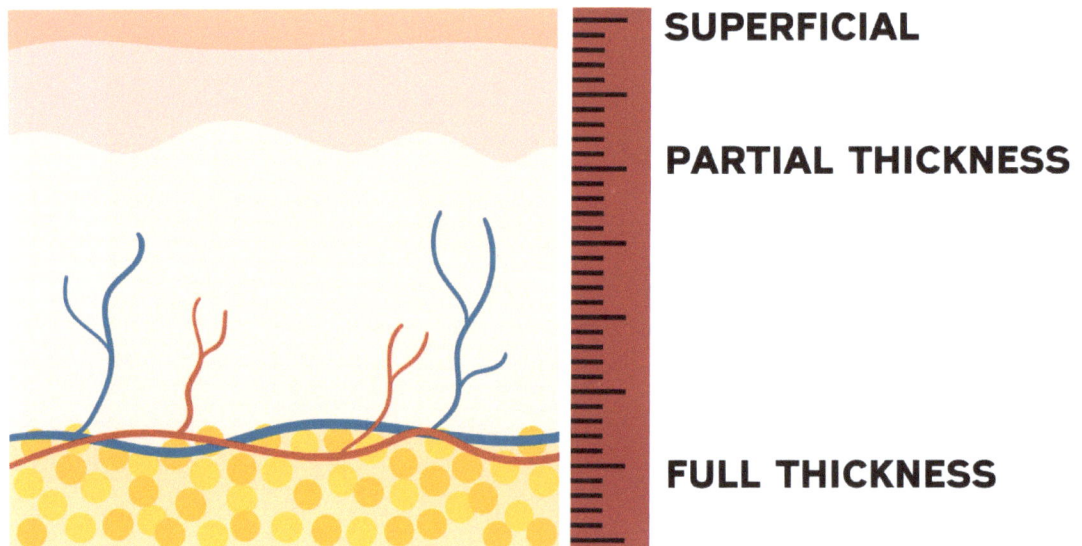

Burn Center Referral[1,3,4]
- Any full-thickness burns
- Partial thickness >10%
- Chemical burns
- Inhalation injury
- Pediatric burns
- Severe facial burns
- Hands, feet, joints, genitals
- Burn-related social resources

Estimating Burn Size[1]

ADULT RULE OF NINES

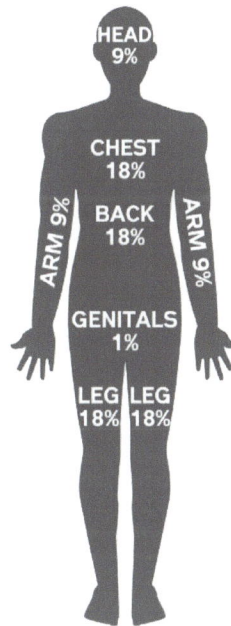

HEAD 9%

CHEST 18%

ARM 9%

BACK 18%

ARM 9%

GENITALS 1%

LEG 18% LEG 18%

PEDIATRIC RULE OF NINES

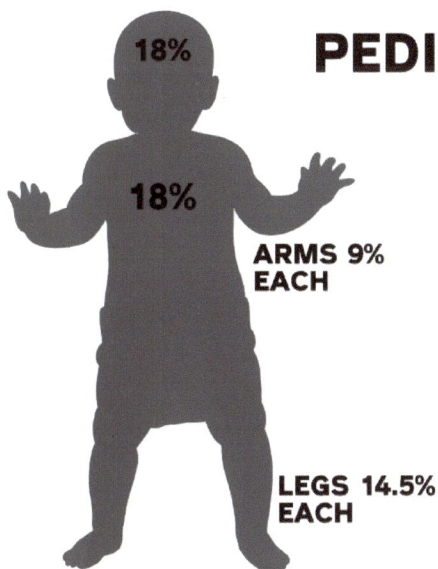

18%

18%

ARMS 9% EACH

LEGS 14.5% EACH

Rule of Palms[1]
It's the PATIENT'S palmar size (fingers included)

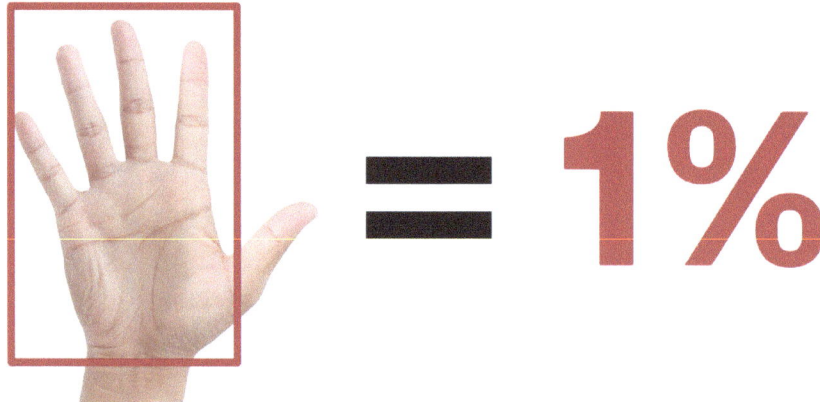

$$= 1\%$$

Inhalation Burns[1,3]
- **Patients may initially appear well**
- **Sympathetic surge prevents airway swelling**
- **Supraglottic injury: severe mucosal edema**
- **Subglottic injury: inflammation, VQ mismatch, pneumonia**
- **INTUBATE EARLY IF ANY SUSPICION OF AIRWAY BURN**

Early Intubation Threshold[1,5]
- **Stridor, hoarseness**
- **Extensive facial burns**
- **Burns inside mouth**
- **Difficulty swallowing**
- **Carbonaceous sputum**
- **Singed nasal hairs**

Toxic Inhalation: Cyanide[1,2]
- **Prevents cell from forming ATP**
- **Initial anxiety and confusion**
- **Initial tachycardia, hypertension**
- **Subsequent total cardiovascular collapse**
- **Wide-gap metabolic acidosis**

Cyanokit[1,2] (hydroxocobalamin)
- May cause temporary reddening of skin
- Side effects
    - Mild hypertension
    - Anxiety
    - N/V
    - Headache
    - Chest discomfort
- Side effects last 2-3 days

Hemoglobin's affinity for carbon monoxide[1]:

CARBON MONOXIDE (CO) **200X** **OXYGEN (O_2)**

Effects of Carbon Monoxide[1,3]

5-10% NORMAL FOR SMOKERS

10-20% HEADACHE, MALAISE

15-40% N/V, MENTAL STATUS CHANGES

>40% SEIZURES, COMA, DEATH

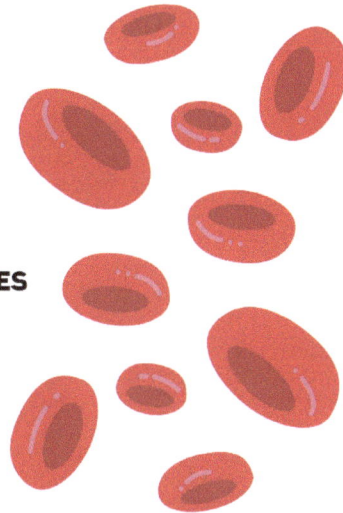

Prehospital Fluid Administration Rate for Burn Patients[1,3,4]
- **>20% total body surface area burned**
- **Partial and full thickness burns only**

ADULTS: age 14+

PEDIATRICS: age 6-13

LITTLE PEDS: age 5 and under

Advanced certification exams continue to test on consensus formula:

2 ML/KG/%BSA → ADULTS WITH THERMALS BURNS

3 ML/KG/%BSA → CHILDREN UNDER 14 YEARS OLD

4 ML/KG/%BSA → KIDS UNDER 30 KG
ALL ELECTRICAL BURNS

Fluid resuscitations is guided by urine output[1,3]

Lactated Ringer's for Burns[1,5]
- **Fluid of choice for burns**
- **Avoid NSS**
- **Blood not recommended**

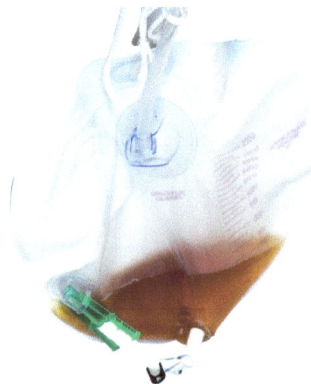

ADULTS: 0.5 ML/KG/HR

PEDS <30KG: 1 ML/KG/HR

HIGH VOLTAGE BURNS: 75-100 ML/HR UNTIL URINE CLEARS

Systemic Burn Response[3,4]
- "Ebb and flow" progression
- Initial low cardiac output state
- 72-96 hours post injury: cardiac output 150% higher
- Markedly high metabolism
  - Increased glucose and O_2 consumption
  - Very high nutritional needs, most patients get TPN
- Cell and capillary damage
  - Inflammation causes severe third-spacing of fluids
- Increased levels of catecholamines, cortisol, and glucagon

Electrical Injury[1,3,5]

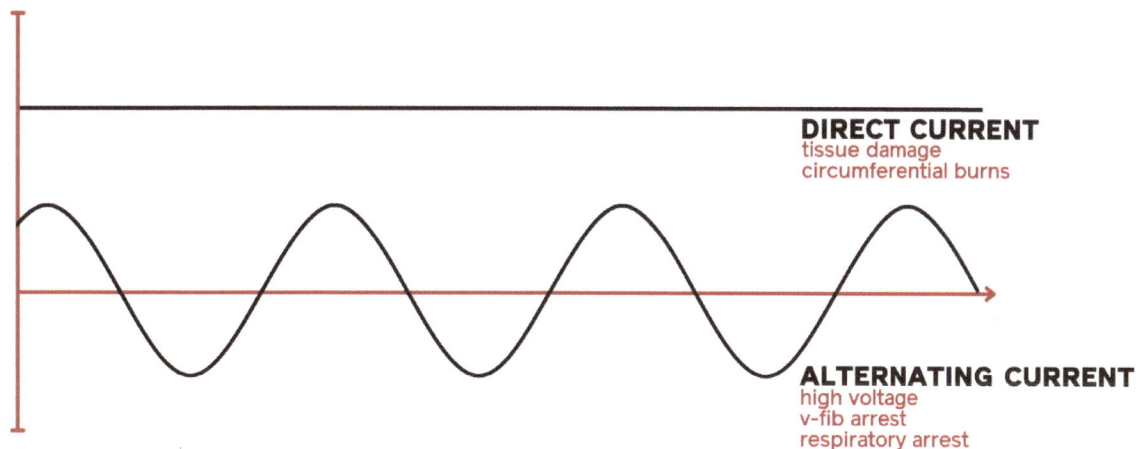

DIRECT CURRENT
tissue damage
circumferential burns

ALTERNATING CURRENT
high voltage
v-fib arrest
respiratory arrest

- Causes circumferential burns
- Arrhythmias
- Nervous tissue conducts electricity
- Muscle destruction causes rhabdo
- Consensus Formula: 4 mL/kg/BSA

Lightening Strikes[1,3]
- Presentation varies
- May cause asystole or V-fib
- Immediate CPR is lifesaving
- Ferning: Lichtenberg Figures

Chemical Burns[1,3]
- Severity is related to:
  - Chemical composition and mech of action
  - Duration of contact
    - BRUSH OFF BEFORE IRRIGATING
  - Quantity of agent
  - Temp of agent
- Alkali: liquify and continue to burn
- Acids: cause coagulative necrosis

Hydrofluoric Acid[3]

- **Even small amounts can cause systemic effects**
- **Severe pain at site of exposure**
- **Systemic hypocalcemia without classic signs**
  - **Eventually cardiovascular effects**
  - **Treat skin with calcium gluconate gel**
  - **IV calcium may be needed**

Escharotomy[1]
- **Not usually recommended for EMS**
- **Indicated in ventilatory compromise**
  - **Decreased air exchange and decreased lung sounds**
  - **Difficulty with ventilation**
    - **Difficult BVM**
    - **High pressures**
  - **Restlessness and agitation**

Radiation Burns[5]

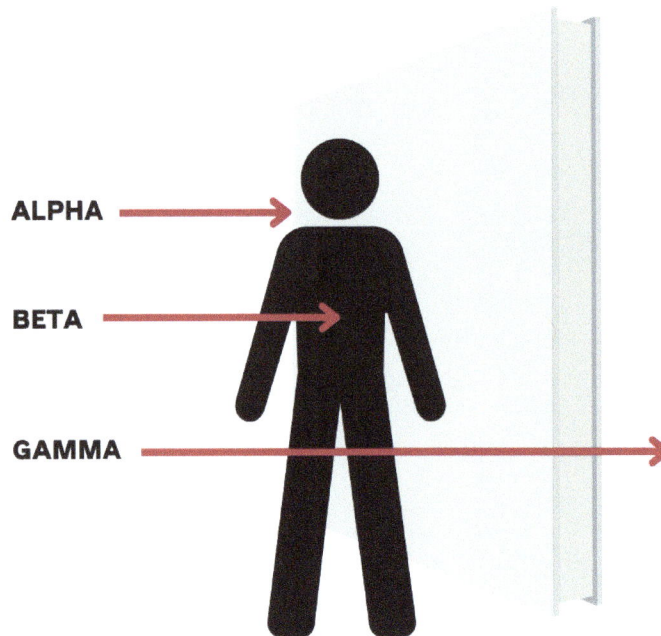

Chapter 13: burns CITATIONS:

1. American Burn Assoc. (2018). ABLS Manual.
2. Desai, Shoma. Su, Mark. (2022). Cyanide Poisoning. Up-to-Date.
3. Feliciano, David V.; Feliciano, David V.; Mattox, Kenneth L.; Mattox, Kenneth L.; Moore, Ernest E.; Moore, Ernest E.. Trauma, Ninth Edition (p. 1058). McGraw Hill LLC. Kindle Edition.
4. Gauglitz, Gerd. Williams, F. (2022). Overview of Complications of Severe Burn Injury. Up-to-Date.
5. Rice, Phillip. Orgill, Dennis. (2022). Emergency Care of Moderate and Severe Thermal Burns in Adults. Up-to-Date.

CHAPTER 14: ENVIRONMENTAL EMERGENCIES

Thermodynamics

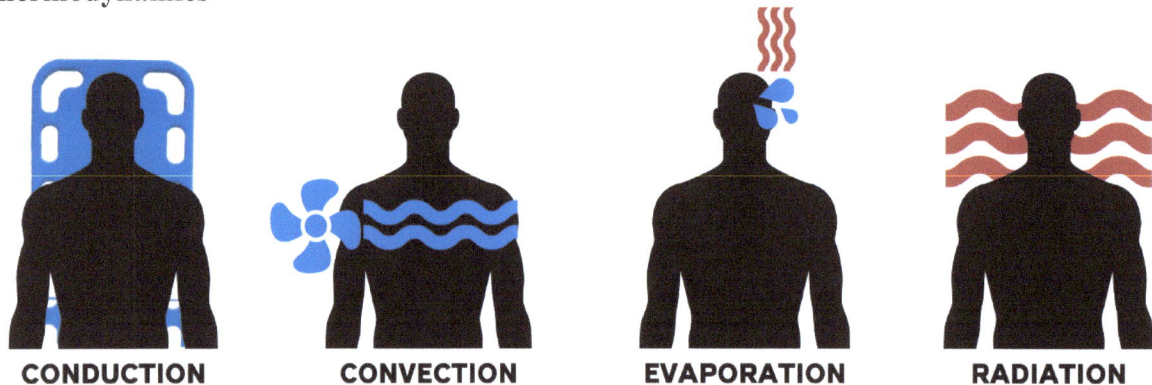

CONDUCTION   CONVECTION   EVAPORATION   RADIATION

THE HYPOTHALAMUS IS THE BODY'S THERMOSTAT

Hypothermia[1]
- **Defined as core temperature < 35ºC (95º F)**
- **Mild: 32º-35ºC**
- **Moderate: 28º-32ºC**
- **Severe: <28ºC**

Hypothermia Initial Presentation[1]
- **Sympathetic response: tachycardia, hyperventilation**
- **Shivering**
- **Ataxia, impaired judgement**
- **Urination ("cold diuresis")**
- **Paradoxical undressing**
- **Atrial fibrillation**

Hypothermia: Later Stages[1]
- **Loss of deep tendon reflexes**
- **Loss of shivering**
- **Hypotension**
- **Bradycardia**
- **Ventricular arrhythmias**
- **Oliguria**

Hypothermia EKG Changes[1]

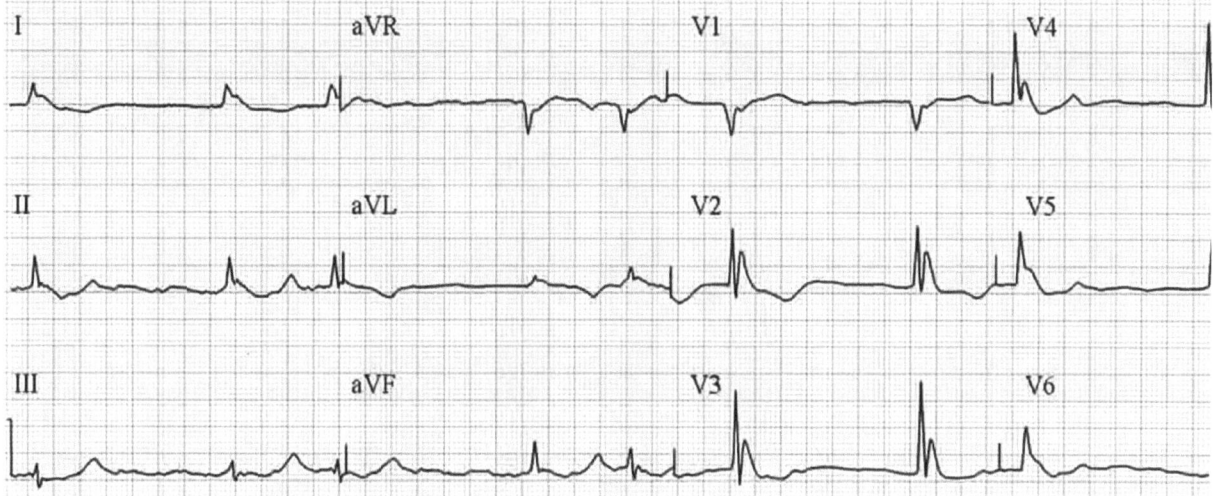

Dead vs. Severe Hypothermia[1]
- CPR is indicated unless the core is frozen and non-compressible
- Rigor is not reliable
- Loss of corneal or pupil reflexes not reliable

Hypothermia Resuscitation[1]
- Check for central pulses for up to 1 minute
  - Extreme bradycardia
- Electricity
  - Defibrillation may be effective
  - Pacing not effective
- Drugs
  - Antiarrhythmics minimally effective
  - Vasopressors are effective
  - ACLS drugs should be given at longer interval

Rewarming[1]
- Passive: mild to moderate
- Active
  - Endovascular temp control catheters
  - Irrigation of thorax or peritoneum
  - ECMO, ECLS, cardiopulmonary bypass

Afterdrop Phenomenon[1]
- Occurs with rewarming
- Acidosis
- Hypotension/vasodilation
- Handle patient with extreme care

Almost Frostbite[2]
- **Frostnip**
- **Chilblains/Pernio**
- **Trench foot**

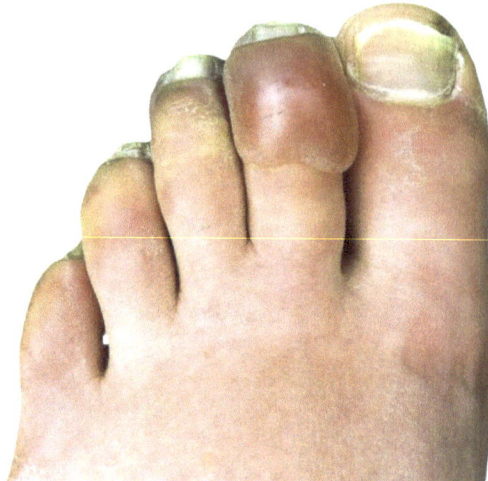

Frostbite[2]
- **Severe, localized cold injury due to freezing of tissue**
- **Remove wet clothing**
- **Splint the extremity**
- **Do not re-warm if ANY potential for re-freezing**
- **Rewarm: immerse in warm water**
- **Possibly TPA for reperfusion**

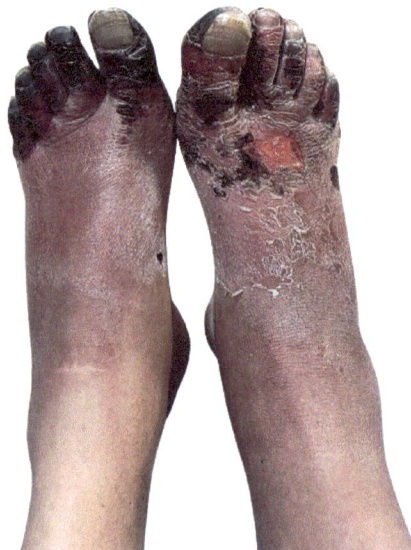

Heat Illness: The Basics[3, 4]
- **Heat cramps: mild**
- **Heat exhaustion: moderate**
- **Heat stroke: severe**

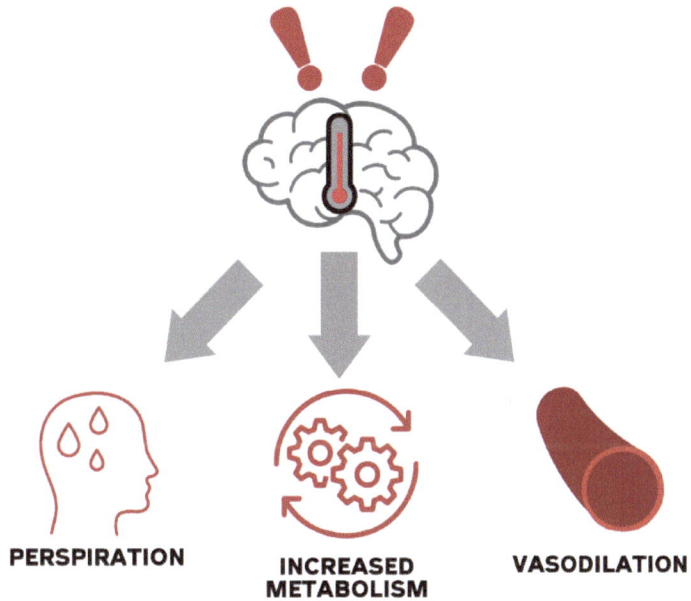

PERSPIRATION   INCREASED METABOLISM   VASODILATION

Heat Stroke[3, 11]
- **Core temp >105ºF**
- **CNS dysfunction**
- **Acute kidney injury**
- **Acute hepatic necrosis**
- **Elevated troponin**
- **Leukocytosis**
- **Rhabdomyolysis**

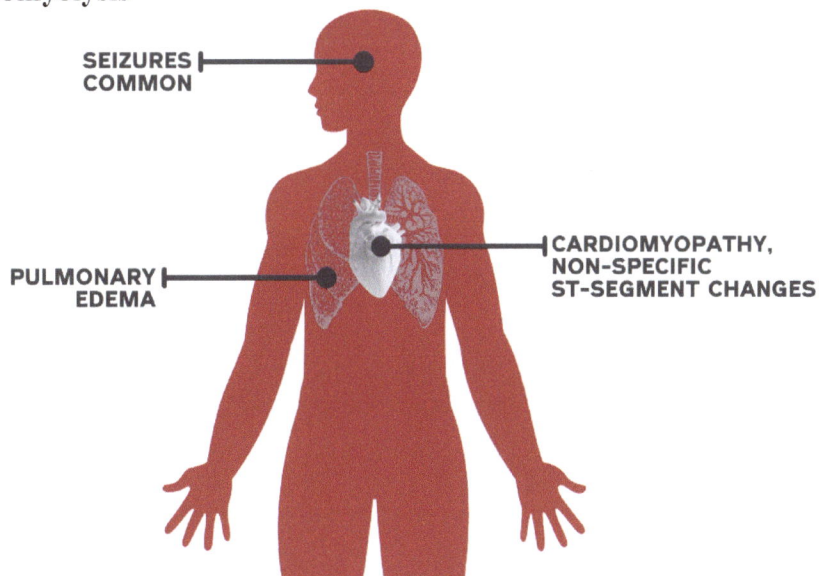

SEIZURES COMMON

PULMONARY EDEMA

CARDIOMYOPATHY, NON-SPECIFIC ST-SEGMENT CHANGES

Heat Illness Treatment[3, 11]
- **Remove from heat, remove clothing, cooling**
- **Cooling temp goal: 38°-39°C**
- **Intubate if AMS**
- **IV access and fluid resuscitation**
- **Benzodiazepines**
- **Dantrolene**

DROWNINGS

Near Drownings[12,13]
- **90% of patients will aspirate some water**
- **Complications of near-drowning events:**
  - **Hypoxia**
  - **V/Q mismatch and shunt**
  - **Direct lung injury**

Salt Water vs. Fresh Water: Doesn't Matter
- **The amount of aspirated water is not enough to make a difference**
- **Need 22 mL/kg for salt-related pathologies**
- **Usual aspirate is 3 mL/kg**

Addressing Drowning Myths
- **Dry drownings are not real**
  - **Monitor 6 hours post near-drowning event**
- **Mammalian Diving Reflex and neuroprotection**
  - **Evidence only supports outcome improvement in extreme hypothermia in the drowning patient**

Prognosticators of poor outcome
- **Greater than 5-minute submersion**
- **Delay in resuscitation**
- **GCS 3 with fixed pupils**
- **pH <7.00**
- **GCS <6 after 8 hours**

ENVENOMATION

Crotalinae[6]
- Thrombin-like enzymes cause coagulation abnormalities
- Fibrin decreases
- Fibrinolysis activated
- Rhabdomyolysis
- Compartment syndrome

Crotalinae Snakebite Syndrome[7]
- Minimal
  - Local, systemic, no coagulopathy
- Moderate
  - Progression of swelling beyond bite site
  - Non-life-threatening symptoms
- Severe
  - Shock
  - Coagulopathy

Pit Viper Bite Treatment
- NO TOURNIQUETS
- Pain control
- Blood products are ineffective

CROFAB[7]
- Crotalidae Polyvalent Immune Fab
- Safe and effective
- Difficult to administer
- Administer in pregnancy

Coral Snakes[5]
- Neurotoxin
- Blocks acetylcholine use at the post-synaptic junction
- Paralysis and cranial nerve palsies
- Respiratory paralysis

Black Widow Spiders[5]
- **Local reaction is usually not problematic**
- **Bites may not cause any issue**
- **Venom contains a-latrotoxin: nerve toxic**
- **Chief symptoms:**
  - **Abdominal pain**
  - **Severe hypertension**
  - **CNS dysfunction – convulsions, muscle spasms**

Brown Recluse Spiders[5]
- **Large ulcers**
- **Expanding tissue necrosis**
- **In rare but severe cases:**
  - **Hemolytic anemia**
  - **Acute renal injury**

Scorpions[5]
- **Blocks neuronal sodium channels**
- **Causes a cholinergic crisis**
- **Severe toxicity is rare but is clinically dramatic**
  - **Fasciculations**
  - **Salivation**
  - **Motor hyperactivity**
  - **Acidosis**
  - **Pulmonary edema**
  - **MODS**
  - **Pancreatitis**

High altitude illness

High Altitude Pathology[8]
- **PO_2 decreases with altitude**
- **Chemoreceptors stimulated by hypoxia:**
  - **Sympathetic stimulation**
  - **Increases minute volume**
  - **Increases cardiac output**
  - **Increased vascular tone**
  - **Increased heart rate**
  - **Increased BP**

High Altitude Cerebral Edema (HACE)
- Primary symptom: altered mental status
- Follows rapid ascent
- May also see:
  - Headache
  - Malaise
  - Ataxia
- Treatment: rapid descent, dexamethasone, oxygen administration/hyperbaric therapy

High Altitude Pulmonary Edema (HAPE)
- Insidious: 2-4 days after ascent
- Most common cause of altitude-related death
- Treated with:
  - Rapid descent
  - Oxygen administration
  - Nifedipine (preventative)
  - Hyperbaric therapy

DIVING EMERGENCIES

Decompression Sickness (DCS)[9,10]
- "The Bends:" musculoskeletal pain (Type 1 DCS)
- "The Chokes:" respiratory (Type 2 DCS)
  - Non-cardiogenic pulmonary edema
  - Results from activation of inflammatory cascade

DCS Manifestations
- Vary widely: may wax and wane, may be static
- 90% are symptomatic within 3 hours of surfacing
- Cutaneous symptoms
- Inner ear pathologies: vertigo, ataxia, tinnitus
- Nitrogen narcosis

Air Embolism
- Symptoms range from mild to catastrophic
- Image: PMID 3443452

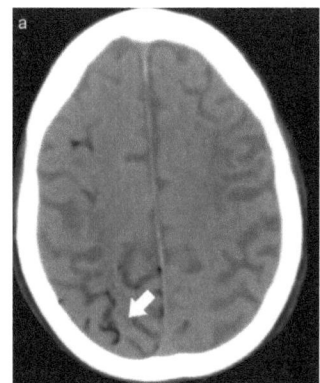

Diving Emergencies Treatment
- Provide 100% oxygen via NRB
- If serious, place patient in horizontal position
- Supportive care

Hyperbaric Oxygen Therapy
- Gold standard in diving related illness therapy
- Provides pure oxygen under pressure
- Enhances removal of nitrogen from the tissues
- Reduces nitrogen bubble sizes
- Safe, low risk

QUESTIONS:

1. The patient with a body temp less than 28 Celsius will present with:

   a. U-waves on EKG
   b. Afterdrop
   c. Absence of shivering
   d. Cold diuresis

Chapter 14 CITATIONS:

1. Zafren, K., Mechem, C., Danzl, D., & Ganetsky, M. (2022, December). Accidental hypothermia in adults. uptodate.com. https://www.uptodate.com/contents/accidental-hypothermia-in-adults

2. Zafren, K., Mechem, C., Danzl, D., & Ganetsky, M. (2022b, December). Frostbite: Emergency care and prevention. uptodate.com. https://www.uptodate.com/contents/frostbite-emergency-care-and-prevention

3. Zafren, K., Mechem, C., Danzl, D., & Ganetsky, M. (2022c, December). Severe nonexertional hyperthermia (classic heat stroke) in adults. uptodate.com. https://www.uptodate.com/contents/severe-nonexertional-hyperthermia-classic-heat-stroke-in-adults

4. Content - Health Encyclopedia - University of Rochester Medical Center. (n.d.). https://www.urmc.rochester.edu/encyclopedia/content.aspx?ContentTypeID=90

5. Sekhon, N. (2019, March). Envenomation. saem.org. https://www.saem.org/about-saem/academies-interest-groups-affiliates2/cdem/for-students/online-education/m4-curriculum/group-m4-environmental/envenomation

6. Ruha, M. (2022https, December). Bites by Crotalinae snakes (rattlesnakes, water moccasins [cottonmouths], or copperheads) in the United States: Management (D. Danzl, S. Traub, & M. Ganetsky, Eds.). uptodate.com. ://www.uptodate.com/contents/bites-by-crotalinae-snakes-rattlesnakes-water-moccasins-cottonmouths-or-copperheads-in-the-united-states-management

7. Sanders, L. (2015, September 11). Management of Venomous Snake Bites in North America. emDOCs.net - Emergency Medicine Education. http://www.emdocs.net/management-of-venomous-snake-bites-in-north-america/

8. Gallagher, S., Hackett, & Rosen, J. (2022, December). High-altitude illness: Physiology, risk factors, and general prevention. uptodate.com. https://www.uptodate.com/contents/high-altitude-illness-physiology-risk-factors-and-general-prevention

9. Sadler, C. (2022). Complications of SCUBA diving. uptodate.com. https://www.uptodate.com/contents/complications-of-scuba-diving

10. Hexdall EJ, Cooper JS. Chokes. [Updated 2022 Dec 4]. In: StatPearls [Internet]. Treasure Island (FL): StatPearls Publishing; 2022 Jan-. Available from: https://www.ncbi.nlm.nih.gov/books/NBK430898/

11. Arleigh Trainor. (2019). Hyperthermia. Available from: https://www.saem.org/about-saem/academies-interest-groups-affiliates2/cdem/for-students/online-education/m4-curriculum/group-m4-environmental/hyperthermia

12. Swaminathan, M., Ellul, M. A., & Cross, T. J. (2018). Hepatic encephalopathy: current challenges and future prospects. Hepatic medicine : evidence and research, 10, 1–11. https://doi.org/10.2147/HMER.S118964

13. Trauma, Burns and Drowning. (n.d.). Deranged Physiology. https://derangedphysiology.com/main/required-reading/trauma-burns-and-drowning

CHAPTER 15: OBSTETRIC EMERGENCIES

CHANGES DURING PREGNANCY

Anatomic & physiologic changes[1]
- **Joints relax**
  - **Progesterone**
- **Gravid uterus encroaches on adjacent structures**
  - **Heart is displaced to the left: left axis deviation on EKG**
    - **Compressions should be performed with this in mind**
  - **Lungs: diaphragm moves up 4cm**
    - **Chest tubes should be inserted one ICS higher**
  - **IVC when laying flat**
  - **Bowel**
  - **Lower extremity circulation**
  - **Renal**
    - **GFR increases 30%**
    - **Increased likelihood of UTI**

Vital Signs
- **Respiratory rate increases**
  - **Minute ventilation increases**
  - **Respiratory alkalosis**
- **Cardiac**
  - **Cardiac output increases 20-30% by 10 weeks gestation, up to 43% by term**
  - **Baseline heart rate increases by 10 beats per minute**
  - **Left axis deviation due to leftward displacement of heart**
  - **Approximate 10mmHg decrease in blood pressure**

Blood volume[1]
- **Circulatory volume increases 40-45% during pregnancy**
  - **Largely plasma**
  - **Dilutional anemia**
- **Pregnant patients will not exhibit clinical signs of hypovolemia until late and severe blood loss**
- **Risk for DVT and PE increases in pregnancy**

Assessment[2]
- **Information**
  - **Number of fetuses**
  - **Gestational age**
  - **LMP**
  - **Estimated due date**
  - **Group B strep status**
  - **Prenatal care**
  - **Known complications**
  - **Complete obstetric history**
  - **Mother's health and social history**

G gravida
Total number of pregnancies

P para
Number of live deliveries

G gravida
Total number of pregnancies

T term
Deliveries at 38+ weeks gestation

P preterm
Deliveries before 37 weeks gestation

A abortions
Pregnancy loss <20 weeks, spontaneous or elective

L living
Number of now living children

Assessment
- **Labor**
  - **Contractions**
  - **Cervical changes**
  - **Membrane**
  - **Intact or ruptured**
  - **Clarity, color, and smell**
  - **Fetal activity**

Cervical changes:
Effacement: cervical thinning, measured in percentage 0-100%
Dilation: cervical opening, measured in centimeters 0-10cm

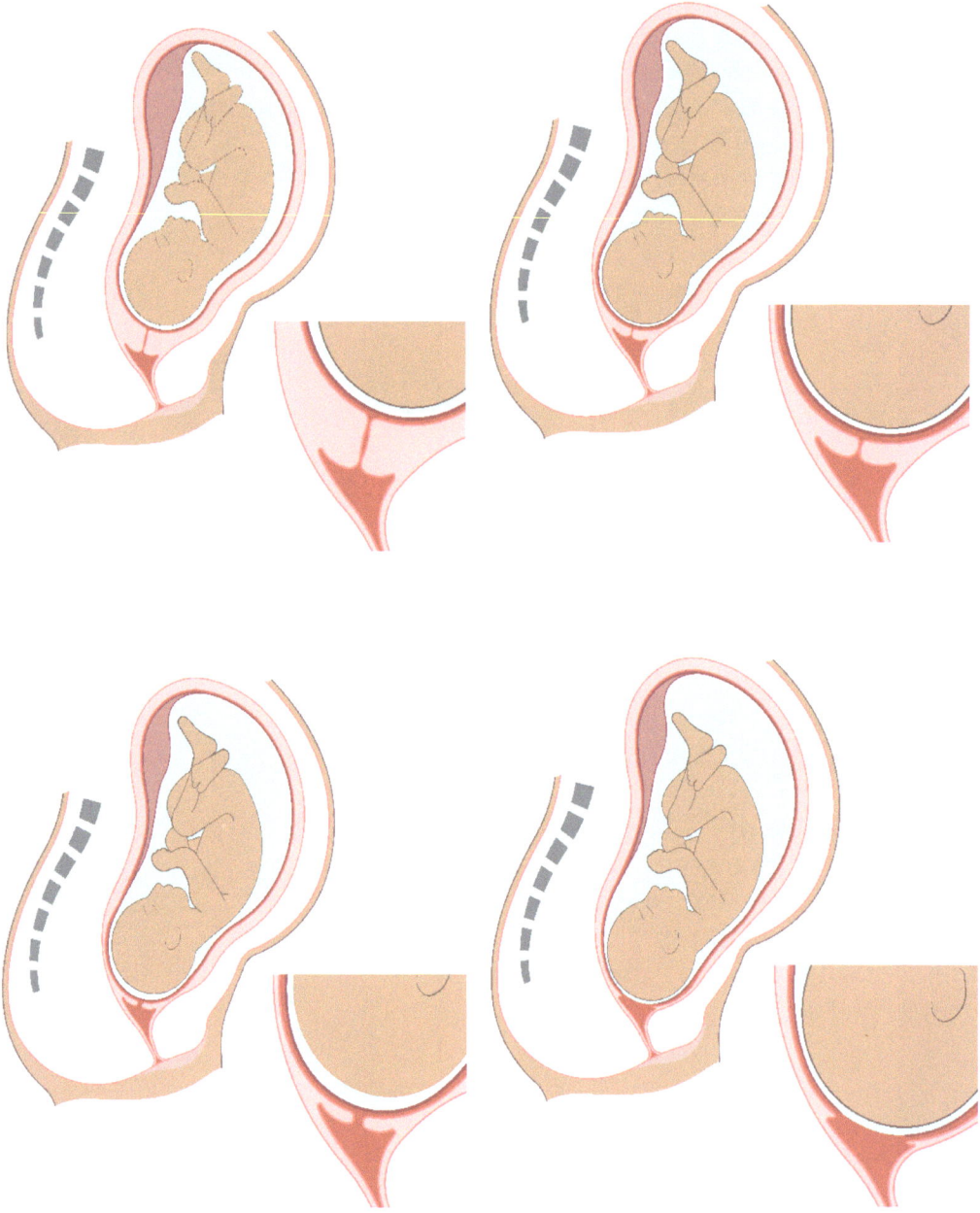

Obstetric practice pearls

- Terminology
    - "spontaneous abortion" vs "miscarriage"
    - Supine hypotension
    - ALWAYS keep mother's pelvis tilted to prevent weight burden of gravid uterus off IVC
- Provider's politics & beliefs: DO NOT let personal beliefs affect rendered care
- If placing a chest tube in gravid patient, go one ICS higher than normal due to upward shift of abdominal and thoracic contents

PREGNANCY COMPLICATIONS

Hyperemesis gravidarum[4]

- Persistent nausea and vomiting
- Leads to dehydration and malnutrition
- Treatment:
    - Assess blood glucose
    - Fluid replacement
    - Antiemetics
    - Reduce visual stimuli

Ectopic pregnancy[5]

- Embryo implants anywhere outside of the uterus
- Symptoms
    - Sudden onset severe abdominal pain
    - Hypovolemic shock
    - Treatment
    - Prehospital: manage blood loss and pain
    - Definitive: methotrexate (early), or surgical

- Hypertension in pregnancy
  One of the leading causes of maternal mortality
- Systolic >140mmHg or Diastolic >90mmHg
    - Two separate readings >6 hours but <7 days apart

HELLP[1]
- **Clinical presentation**
    - **Can lead to MODS**
    - **Presents with RUQ pain and malaise**
    - **15% of cases will not have hypertension or proteinuria**
    - **Treatment**
    - **Blood product administration**
    - **Magnesium and antihypertensives**
    - **Delivery of fetus & placenta**

Hemolytic anemia,

Elevated

Liver enzymes,

Low

Platelet count

Pre-eclampsia[1]
- **Clinical presentation**
    - **Hypertension**
    - **Proteinuria**
    - **Hyperreflexia**
    - **Edema**
    - **Abdominal pain**
- **Treatment**
    - **IV magnesium bolus 4-6 grams over 20 minutes**
    - **IV magnesium drip 2-4 grams per hour**
    - **IV labetalol, hydralazine, or nifedipine**
    - **Delivery of fetus & placenta**

Eclampsia[1]
- **New onset seizures with pre-eclampsia or HELLP**
- **First line treatment: magnesium bolus and drip**
- **Transport priority: prevent seizures**

Magnesium complications

- **Magnesium toxicity**
    - **Symptoms: loss of DTR, respiratory depression, AMS**
    - **Treatment: calcium gluconate or calcium chloride**
    - **Mag exposed baby**
    - **Lethargic**
    - **Higher likelihood of need for resuscitation**

Placenta previa[1,2]
- **Placental implantation near or over the cervical opening**
- **Presents as painless bright red vaginal bleeding**
- **Transport priorities**
    - **Vaginal exam is contraindicated**
    - **Maintain maternal hemodynamic stability**
    - **Transport to HROB center for cesarean section**

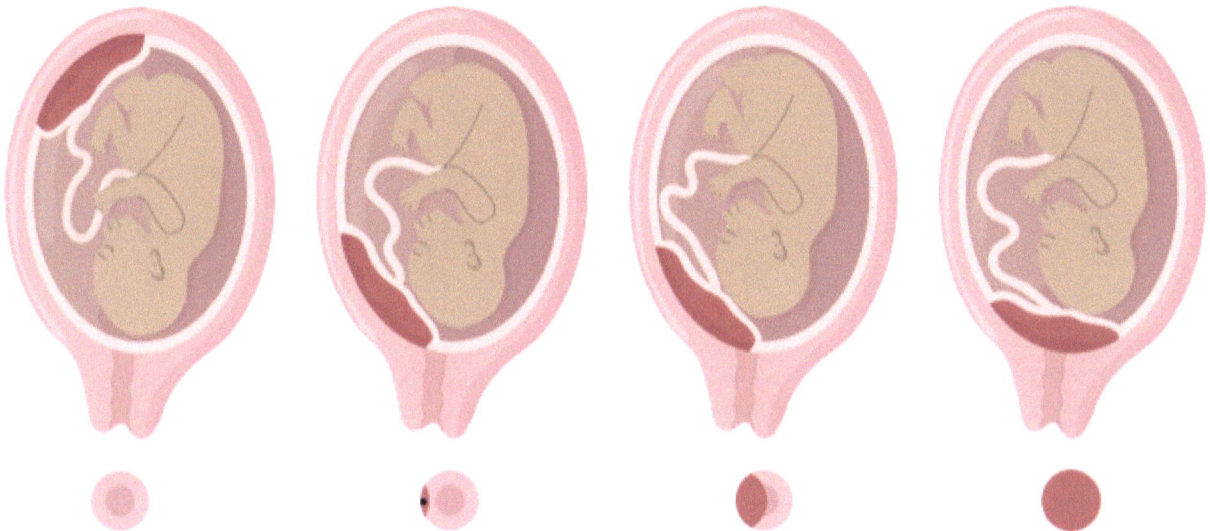

Placental abruption[1,2,5]
- **Separation of a normally positioned placenta from uterine wall**
- **Clinical presentation**
    - **Sudden onset painful bleeding* with radiation to the back**
    - **Decreased fetal movement and heart tones**
    - **Hypovolemic shock**
    - **Rigid uterus, tender abdomen**

*Bleeding can present externally or remain concealed inside the uterus

Pre-term labor[2]

- Labor between 20w and 37w6d gestation
- Treatment
  - Tocolytics
    - Terbutaline: contraindicated in patients with cardiac history
    - Nifedipine
    - Indomethacin: contraindicated past 32 weeks gestation
  - Corticosteroids: short term use to achieve lung maturity or for transport to HROB center with NICU capabilities

Premature rupture of membranes (PROM)[2]

- Spontaneous rupture of amniotic sac before 37 weeks
- Treatment*
  - Delivery within 24 hours

  -OR-
  - Hospitalization with IV antibiotics until delivery

  In the case of full rupture; there can be small leaks that spontaneously resolve

Gestational diabetes[1]

- Pregnancy-induced hormone changes can alter insulin effectiveness and cause gestational diabetes
- Treatment
  - Dietary changes
  - Insulin therapy
  - Delivery

Missed abortion/retained products

- The body attempts to rid the uterus of these products of conception with heavy bleeding
- Assess the number of pads saturated with blood per hour, anything >1 per hour is concerning
- Treatment
  - Prehospital: maintain hemodynamic stability
  - Definitive: dilation and curettage (D&C)

COMPLICATIONS OF DELIVERY

Maternal fever
- Intrapartum fever >100.4°F or 38°C
- Increases likelihood of neonatal sepsis and hypoxic birth injuries
- Treat with antipyretics

Group B streptococcus (GBS)
- Maternal testing at 35 weeks gestation
- Requires initial dose of IV penicillin during labor, plus Q4 hour ongoing dosing through active labor
- If not administered during labor (fast labor, out of hospital delivery, etc.), baby will require prophylactic treatment

Breech presentation
- DO NOT APPLY TRACTION TO PRESENTING PART
- If shoulders become entrapped, rotate fetus to one shoulder at the 12 o'clock position[1]
- Once arms have delivered, rotate fetus so baby's face is toward mother's posterior
  - Place two fingers into vagina to hold vaginal wall off baby's nose

Shoulder dystocia
- Head delivers but shoulders impinge on pelvis
- Turtle sign: when the shoulder dystocia applies traction to pull head back toward uterus
- Treatment: McRoberts maneuver
  - Flex mother's knees against her chest during next contraction
  - Apply <u>suprapubic</u> pressure to fold baby's shoulders inward to allow for passage under pubic symphysis (NOT fundal pressure)

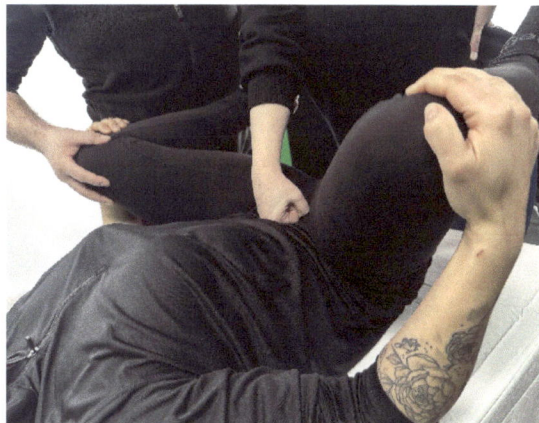

Umbilical cord prolapse
- Umbilical cord presents before fetus
- Treatment
    - Hold presenting part off cervix and cord
    - Place mother on 100% oxygen by nonrebreathing mask
    - Position mother on all fours with knees to chest, hips above shoulders

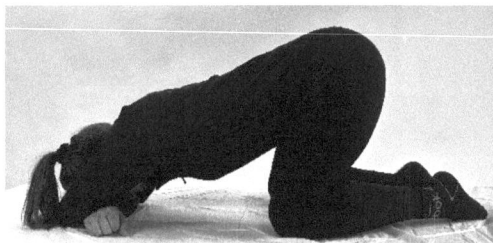

Nuchal cord
- Low incidence of complications
- Easily resolved by pulling loop back over baby's head

En caul delivery
- Neonate is delivered with amniotic sac intact
- Rare, but more common in pre-term deliveries
- Treatment: Rupture membranes after delivery

Post-partum hemorrhage[5]
- Blood loss >500mL within 24 hours of delivery
- Identify and treat provocative factors
    - Lacerations: apply direct pressure to external lacerations, suture repair by physician
    - Retained products: D&C
    - Uterine atony: IV Pitocin, fundal massage, place baby to breast
    - REBOA in zone 3 to OR
    - Manage hemodynamic stability with blood administration

Cardiac arrest in pregnancy[3]
- Causes: trauma, amniotic fluid embolism, peripartum cardiomyopathy, severe hypertension
- Amniotic fluid embolism: small amount of amniotic fluid enters maternal circulation and induces anaphylactoid reaction
  - Treat with A-OK (Atropine, Ondansetron, Ketorolac)
- Treatment: provide ongoing resuscitation attempts and rapid transport to capable facility for perimortem cesarean section

Rh compatibility
- Rh negative mother carrying Rh positive fetus
  - Production in maternal antibody to Rh factor
  - Affects subsequent pregnancies
  - Treatment: IM Rhogam at 28 weeks and delivery, or at time of pregnancy loss

Delivery pearls
- Expect placental delivery up to 30 minutes after neonate
  - Do not apply traction to umbilical cord
- Prioritize skin to skin contact if patients are stable
  - Prevents neonatal hypothermia
- Breastfeeding prevents neonatal hypoglycemia
  - Encourages placental delivery
  - Prevents post-partum hemorrhage

Fetal assessment and heart monitoring

Assessment[2]
- Fetal position
  - Head and buttocks can be palpated
- Fetal heart monitoring
  - Doppler fetal heart tones every 15 minutes
  - Tocodynamometer if available

Fetal heart monitoring[2]
- Fetal heart rate and patterns are used to assess oxygenation status and the presence of distress
  - Normal fetal heart rate: 110-160 beats per minute
  - Fetal tachycardia
    - Compensates for transient hypoxia
    - Maternal fever
  - Fetal bradycardia indicates fetal compromise[1]
    - Cord compression
    - Placental insufficiency
    - Maternal hypotension
    - Uterine rupture

- Variability
  - Fluctuations from baseline
  - Absent: no variability, associated with fetal distress
  - Minimal: 0-5 bpm variability
  - Moderate: 6-25 bpm variability
  - Marked: >25 bpm variability
- Acceleration
  - Indicates fetal movement or stimulation
  - Increase in fetal heart rate >15 bpm lasting >15 seconds

Fetal heart monitoring: Decelerations[2]
- <u>Early decelerations</u>: mirror contraction, normal during active labor, indicates head compression
- <u>Variable decelerations</u>: abrupt decrease in fetal HR, characterized by v- or w-shapes
  - Indicates cord compression or compromise
  - Treatment: change maternal position, fluid administration, 100% oxygen, tocolysis
- <u>Late decelerations</u>: nearly symmetrical with contraction, but begins and returns to baseline after the contraction ends
  - Indicates placental insufficiency
  - Requires immediate intervention

Sinusoidal Pattern
- Indicates impending fetal demise
- High rate of fetal morbidity and mortality

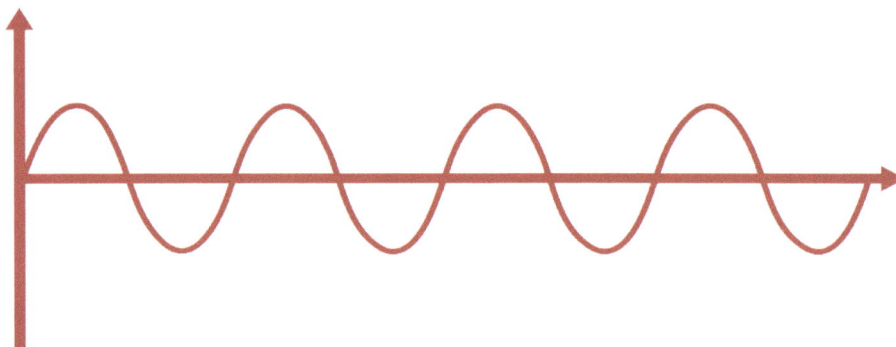

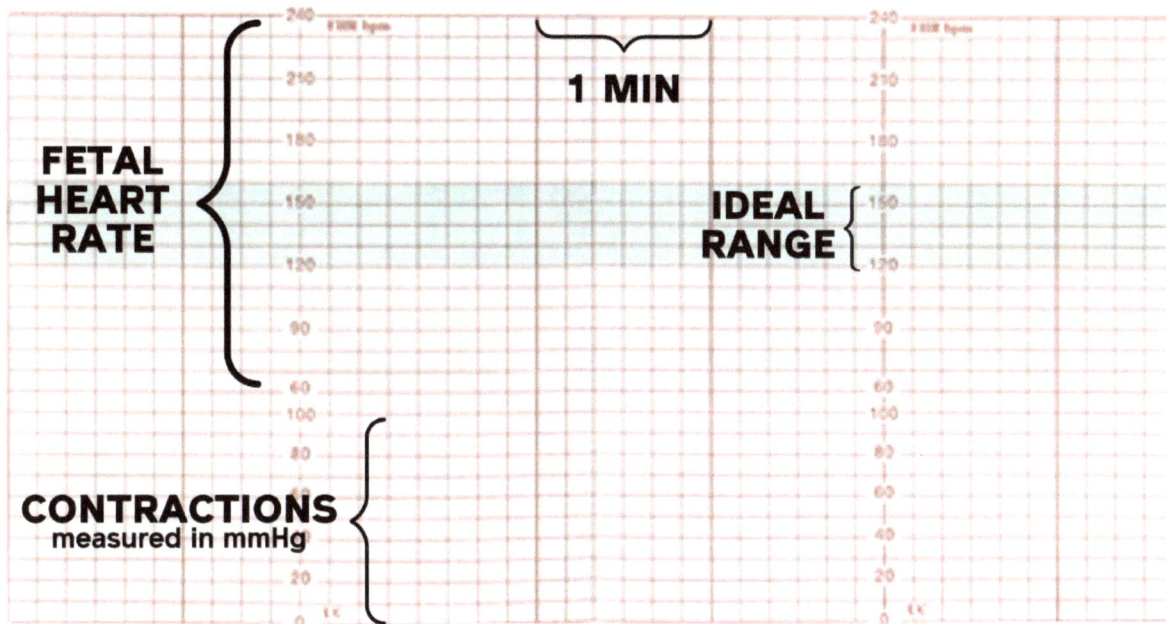

FETAL
HEART
RATE

1 MIN

IDEAL
RANGE

CONTRACTIONS
measured in mmHg

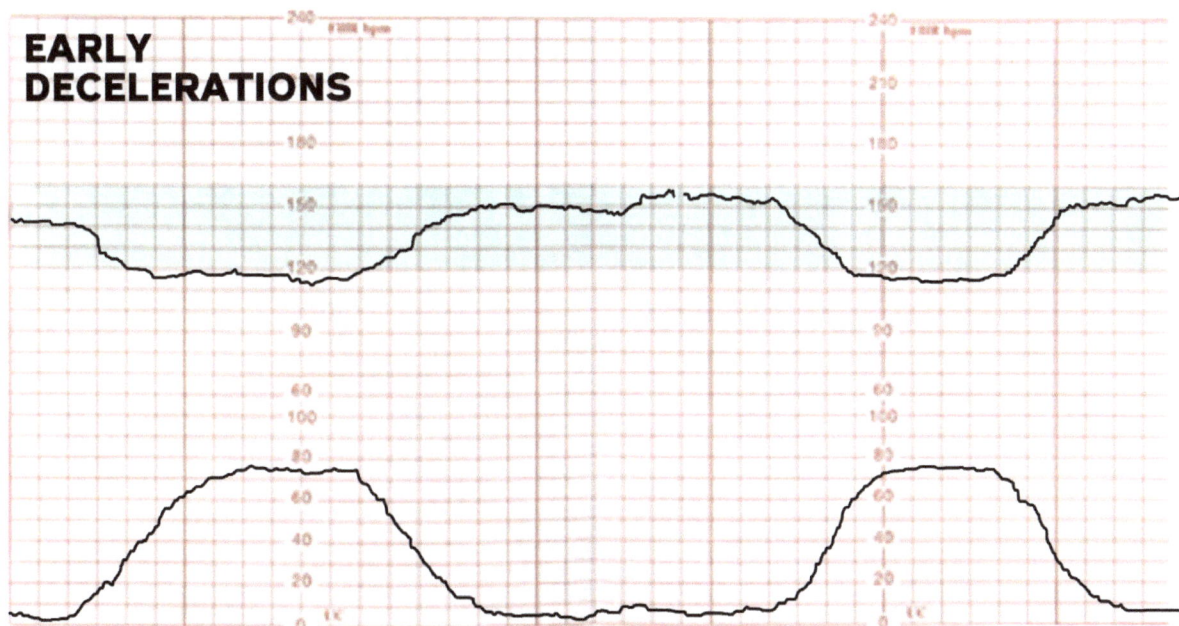

EARLY
DECELERATIONS

LATE
DECELERATIONS

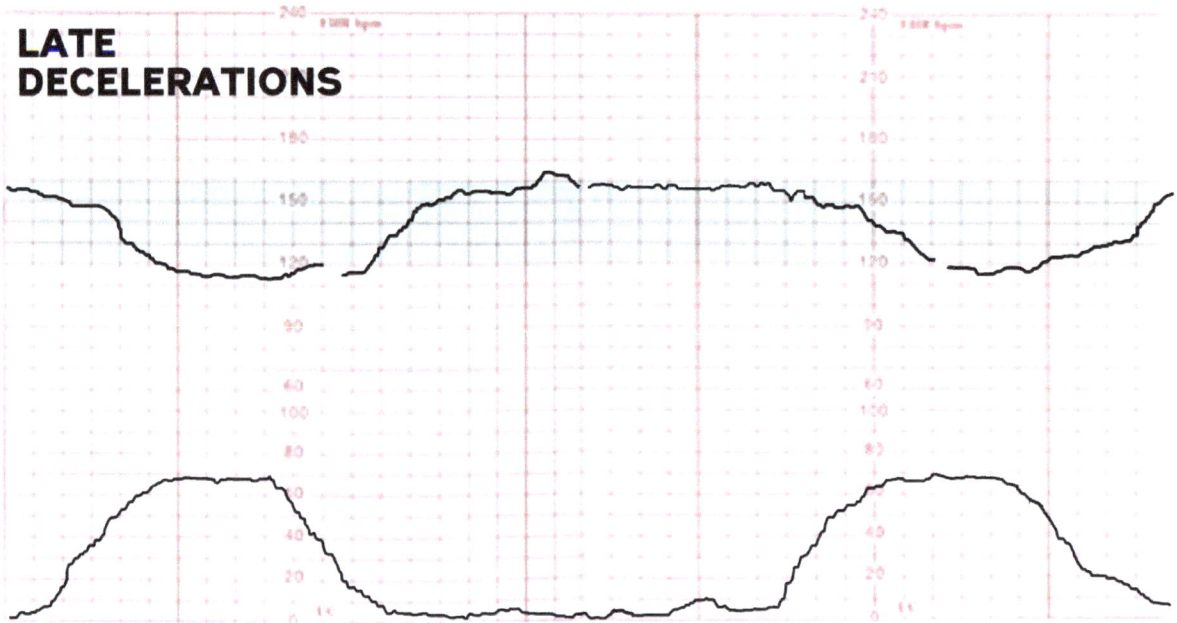

VARIABLE
DECELERATIONS

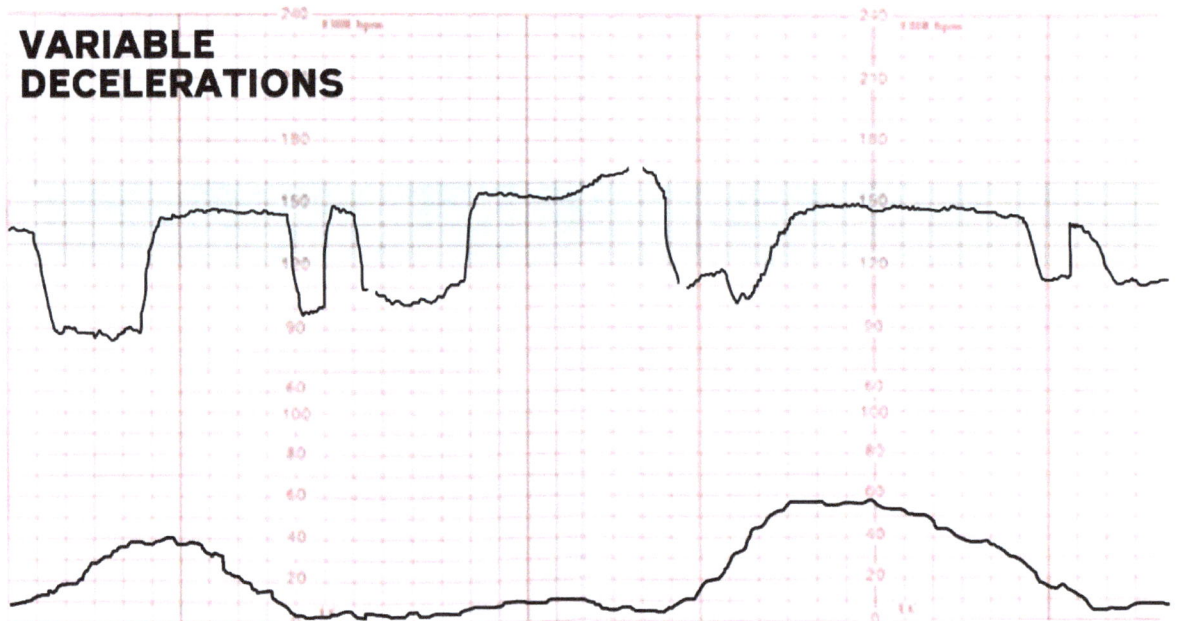

ACCELERATIONS

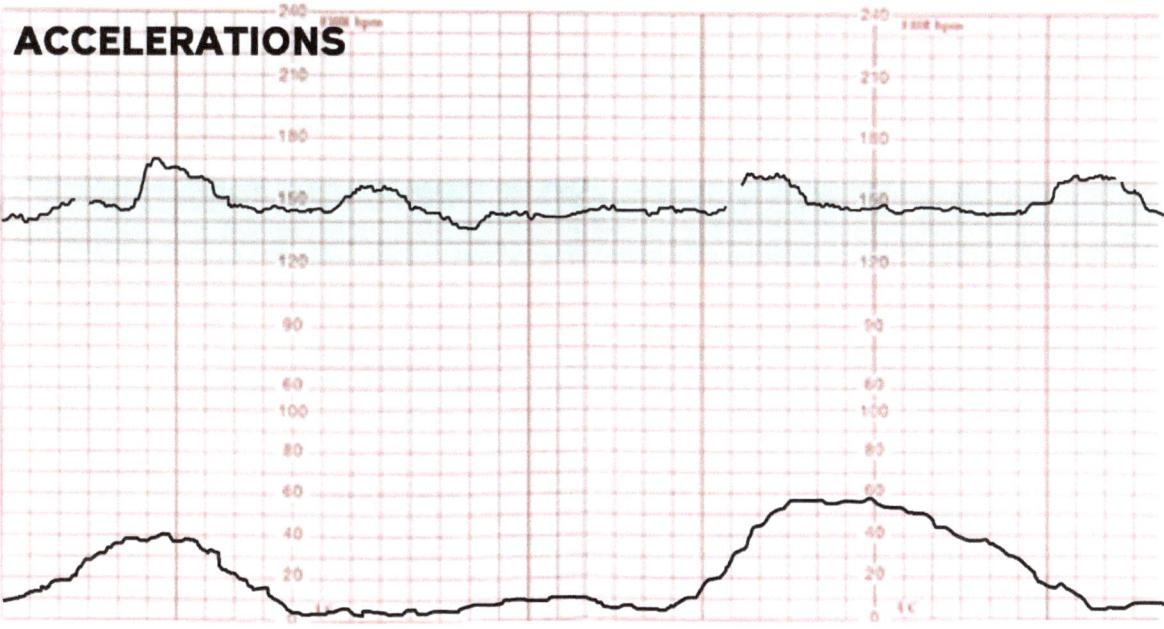

**SINUSOIDAL FETAL
HEART TRACING**

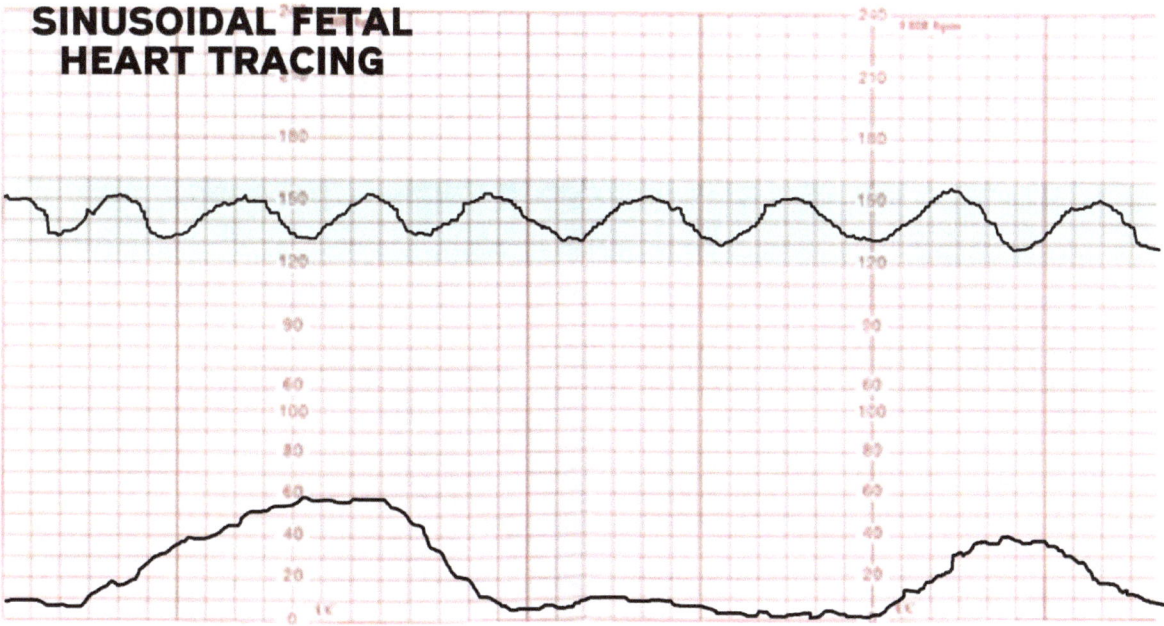

VARIABLE DECELERATION
ABRUPT DECREASE OF >15BPM LASTING 15-120 SECONDS

CORD COMPRESSION
CONTRACTION, NUCHAL CORD, CORD PROLAPSE, TRUE KNOT

EARLY DECELERATION
MIRRORS SHAPE AND TIMING OF CONTRACTION

HEAD COMPRESSION
DUE TO VAGAL STIMULATION OF FETUS BY CONTRACTION

ACCELERATION
ABRUPT INCREASE >15BPM LASTING >15 SECONDS

OKAY
THIS IS AN EXPECTED AND NORMAL FINDING

LATE DECELERATION
DELAYED PAST THE START AND FINISH OF CONTRACTION

PLACENTAL INSUFFICIENCY
COMPROMISE IN PLACENTAL PERFUSION

Neonatal care
- 90-95% of live births require no medical intervention
- It takes up to 10 minutes for neonate to reach SpO_2 >90%
- Warm and dry neonate, discard wet towel
- Suction should only be performed if PPV given
- APGAR scores at 1- and 5-minutes post birth

	0	1	2
Appearance	blue and pale	body pink, limbs blue	all pink
Pulse	absent	<100	>100
Grimace	no response	grimace	cough and crying
Activity	limp	weak	strong
Respirations	absent	irregular, slow	strong cry

questions:

1. You are requested to transport a 28-year-old female G3P2 35w4d who is having regular contractions and is 100%/4cm from a small hospital with OB services but without NICU capabilities to a HROB/Level 4 NICU 40 minutes away by rotor. The patient has had a mag bolus and is currently on a mag drip at 4g/hr. Your priority is:

    a. Plan for ground transport
    b. Increase mag drip to 6g/hr
    c. Administer calcium gluconate
    d. Load and go (by rotor)

2. You are working 911 and respond to a call of a 15-year-old female 37w6d at her home. She reports her water broke about 30 minutes ago and that her back is in excruciating pain. Complications to expect if you delivery this neonate during transport should include:

    a. HELLP syndrome
    b. Breech delivery
    c. Post partum hemorrhage
    d. Shoulder dystocia

3. You are transporting a 39w2d 30-year-old female from a rural facility without OB services to an appropriate facility 15 minutes by rotor after rendezvousing with a ground crew. You place the patient on toco and see the following strip.

    What interventions would you perform?

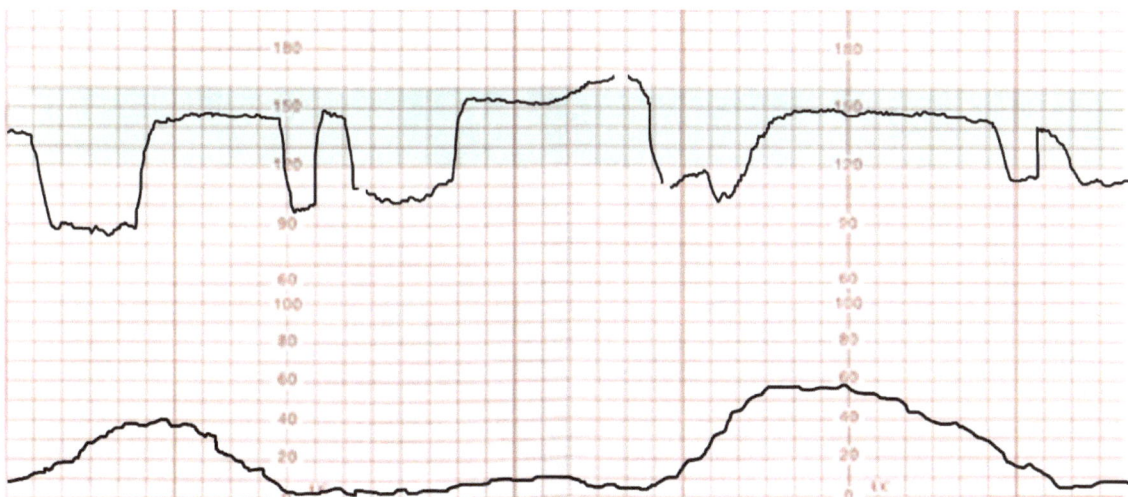

Chapter 15 citations:

1. Mejia, A. (2022). Critical Care Transport (3rd ed.). Jones and Bartlett Learning.
2. Air & Surface Transport Nurses Association, & Clark, D. J. Y. S. (2017). Critical Care Transport Core Curriculum. Air & Surface Transport Nurses Association.
3. Pregnancy Mortality Surveillance System | Maternal and Infant Health | CDC. (n.d.). https://www.cdc.gov/reproductivehealth/maternal-mortality/pregnancy-mortality-surveillance-system.htm
4. Caroline, N. L. & American Academy of Orthopaedic Surgeons (AAOS). (2017). Nancy Caroline's Emergency Care in the Streets (8th ed.). Jones & Bartlett Learning.

Chapter 16: Neonatal emergencies and transport

Neonatal Terminology
- <u>Newborn:</u> an infant within the first few hours of birth
- <u>Neonate:</u> an infant within the first 28 days of birth
- <u>Term Newborn:</u> an infant delivered in the 37th to 42nd week of gestation
- <u>Pre-Term Newborn:</u> an infant delivered prior to the 37th week of gestation

Normal Neonatal Vital Signs

	Weight in lbs	Weight in kgs	Resp Rate	Heart Rate	Systolic BP
Preterm (<37 wks)	1.5-5.5	0.7-2.5	50-70	120-180	40-60
Newborn (37-42 wks)	5.5-9	2.5-4	40-60	100-170	50-70
Neonate (1-28 days)	7.5-11	3.4-5	30-50	90-160	60-80
Infant (1-12 months)	10-22	4.5-10	25-40	80-160	70-100
Toddler (1-3 years)	22-32	10-14.5	20-30	80-130	70-110
Preschooler (3-5 years)	32-42	14.5-19	20-30	80-110	80-110
School Age (6-12 years)	42-90	19-41	20-24	75-100	80-120
Adolescent (>13 years)	>90	>41	12-20	60-90	94-130

Neonatal Anatomy & Physiology

Thermoregulation[2]

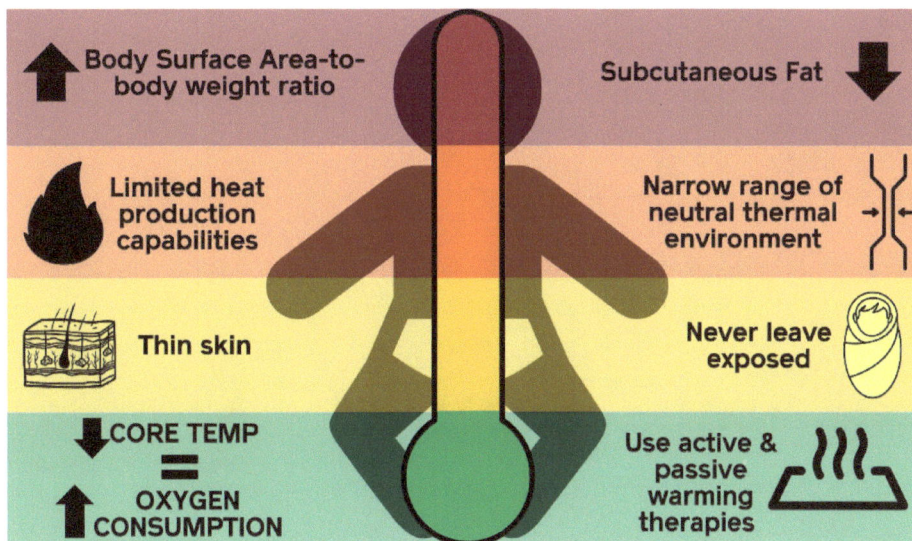

Pulmonary System[1]

- Lung development is unable to sustain life at <23 weeks gestation or <1lb of fetal weight
- Full term neonatal tidal volume of 5-7 mL/kg
- At birth lungs are filled with fluid
  - Within 10 seconds, neonatal CNS senses new environment and the infant will gasp

Physiologic Changes at Birth[4]

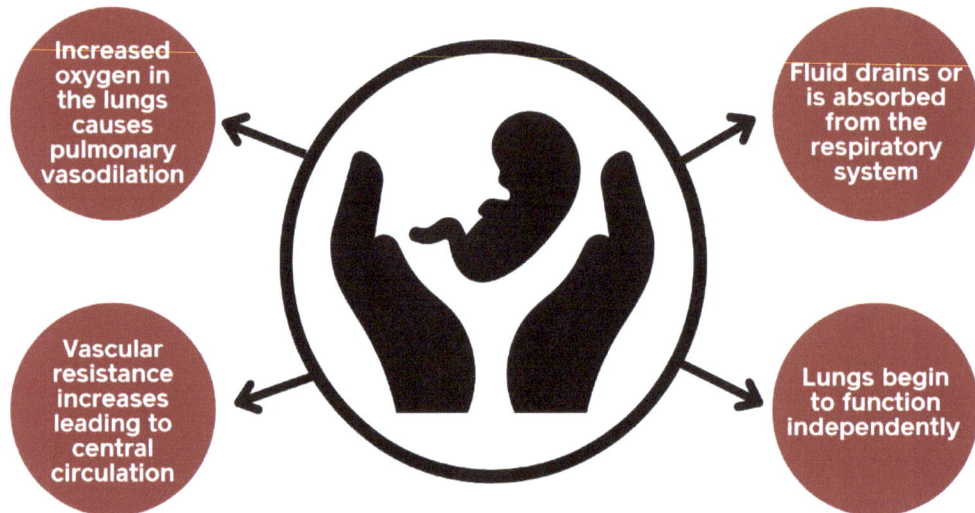

Increased oxygen in the lungs causes pulmonary vasodilation

Fluid drains or is absorbed from the respiratory system

Vascular resistance increases leading to central circulation

Lungs begin to function independently

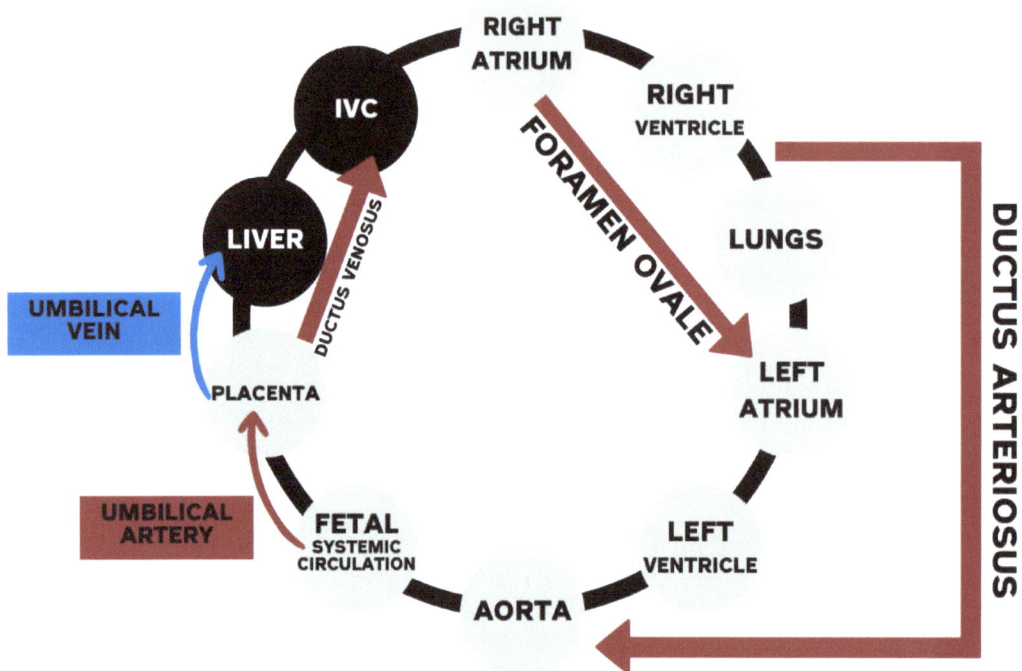

RIGHT ATRIUM

RIGHT VENTRICLE

IVC

LUNGS

FORAMEN OVALE

LIVER

DUCTUS VENOSUS

UMBILICAL VEIN

LEFT ATRIUM

PLACENTA

DUCTUS ARTERIOSUS

UMBILICAL ARTERY

FETAL SYSTEMIC CIRCULATION

LEFT VENTRICLE

AORTA

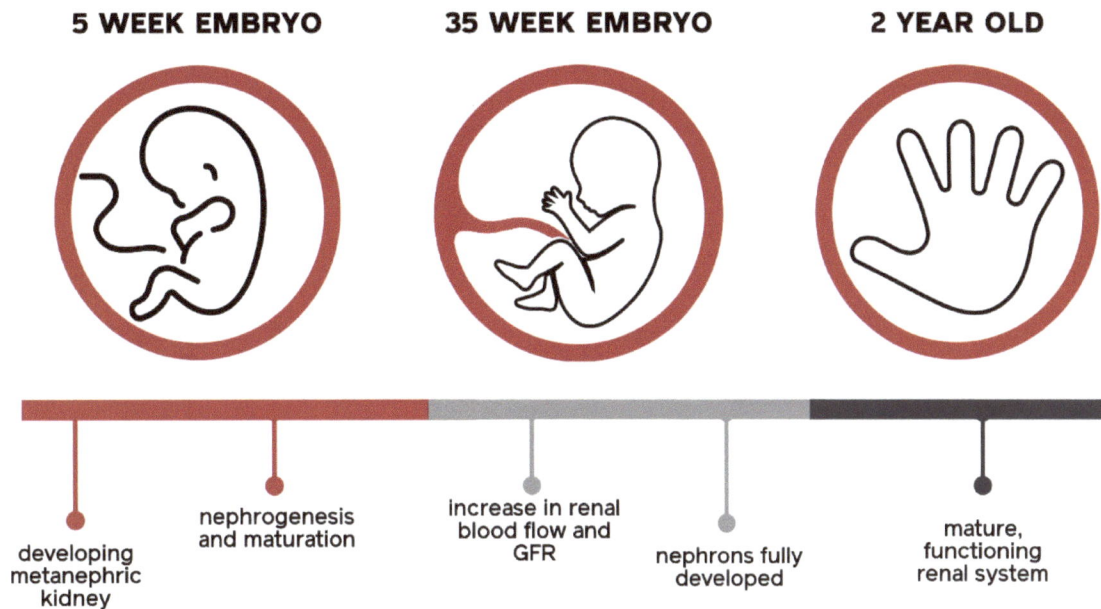

5 WEEK EMBRYO **35 WEEK EMBRYO** **2 YEAR OLD**

developing metanephric kidney

nephrogenesis and maturation

increase in renal blood flow and GFR

nephrons fully developed

mature, functioning renal system

Neonatal assessment & Intervention

Primary Assessment[7]

- **Term assessment**
  - **Does the neonate appear to be full term vs. pre-term**
- **Tone**
  - **Limp vs. vigorous**
- **Respiratory effort**
  - **Breathing/crying vs. silent/apneic**

	0	1	2
Appearance	blue and pale	body pink, limbs blue	all pink
Pulse	absent	<100	>100
Grimace	no response	grimace	cough and crying
Activity	limp	weak	strong
Respirations	absent	irregular, slow	strong cry

APGAR should be performed at 1 and 5 minutes after delivery

NEONATAL RESUSCITATION FOR PREHOSPITAL

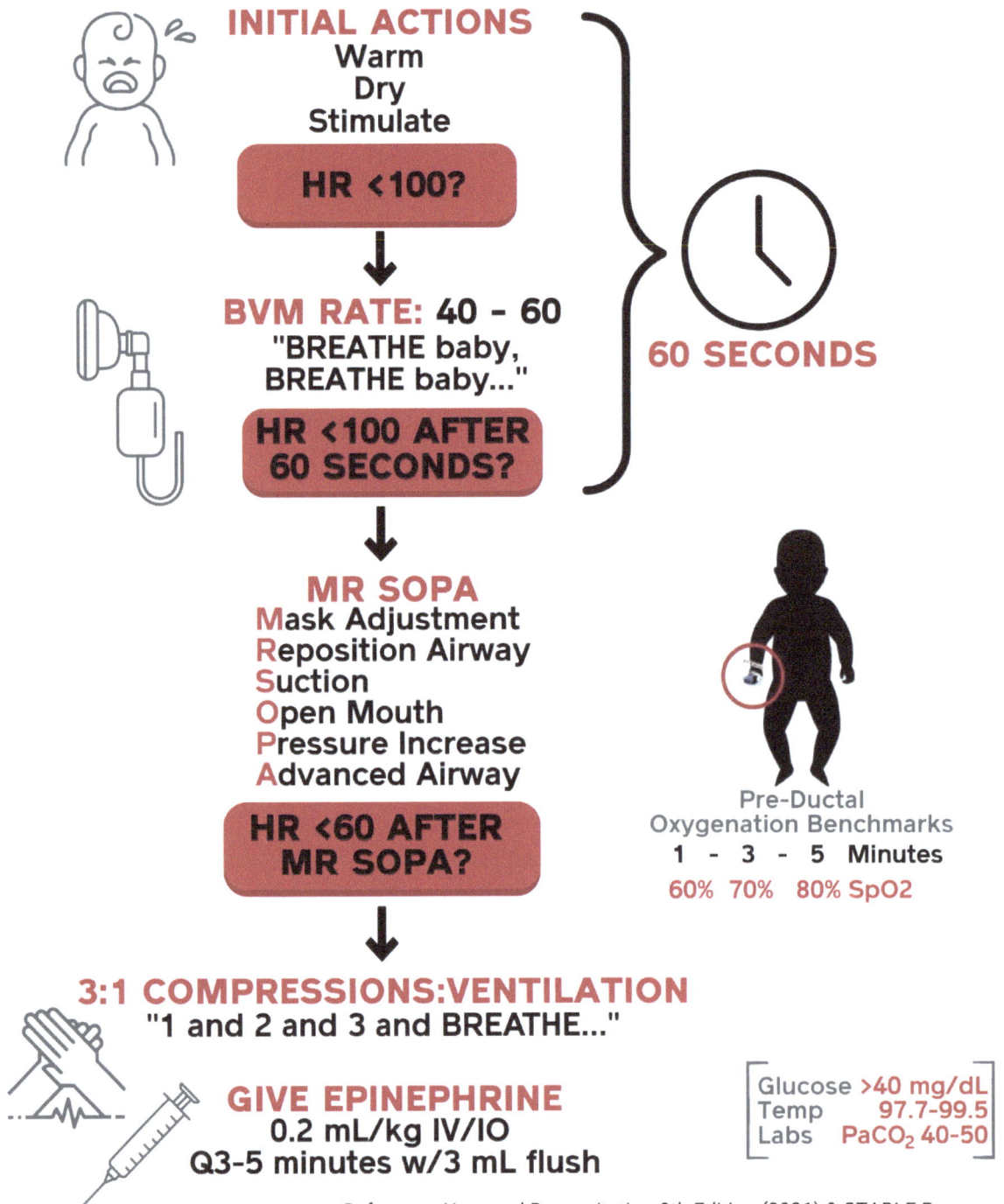

INITIAL ACTIONS
Warm
Dry
Stimulate

HR <100?

BVM RATE: 40 - 60
"BREATHE baby,
BREATHE baby..."

**HR <100 AFTER
60 SECONDS?**

60 SECONDS

MR SOPA
Mask Adjustment
Reposition Airway
Suction
Open Mouth
Pressure Increase
Advanced Airway

**HR <60 AFTER
MR SOPA?**

Pre-Ductal
Oxygenation Benchmarks
1 - 3 - 5 Minutes
60% 70% 80% SpO2

3:1 COMPRESSIONS:VENTILATION
"1 and 2 and 3 and BREATHE..."

GIVE EPINEPHRINE
0.2 mL/kg IV/IO
Q3-5 minutes w/3 mL flush

Glucose >40 mg/dL
Temp   97.7-99.5
Labs   PaCO$_2$ 40-50

Reference: Neonatal Resuscitation 8th Edition (2021) & STABLE Program

Stabilization and Treatment
- **Suction**
  - **Mouth, then nose**
  - **Bulb syringe, 10F or 14F catheter**
  - **CPAP if peripheral cyanosis* despite adequate respiratory effort**
  - **PEEP 4-6 cmH$_2$O**

Takes up to 10 minutes to reach SpO$_2$ of 90-100%

Free-Flow Oxygen
- **Ineffective in neonate with poor ventilatory effort**
  - **Use PPV**
  - **Oxygen should be warmed and humidified**
  - **Caution: long term oxygen use causes many complications**
- **If PPV is not needed, deliver via simple mask**

Continuous Positive Airway Pressure (CPAP)
- **First line ventilatory support in neonates**
  - **PEEP 4-6 cmH$_2$O**
  - **Room air for full term neonates**
  - **30-100% FiO$_2$ for preterm neonates**
  - **Expected full term neonatal SpO$_2$: 95-98%**
- **Expected preterm neonatal SpO$_2$: 88-92%**

Neonatal Intubation

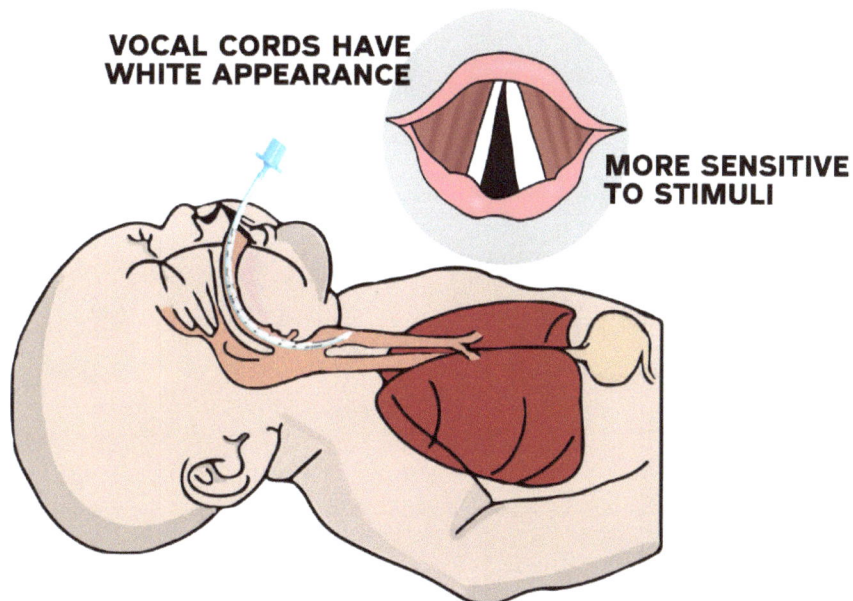

VOCAL CORDS HAVE WHITE APPEARANCE

MORE SENSITIVE TO STIMULI

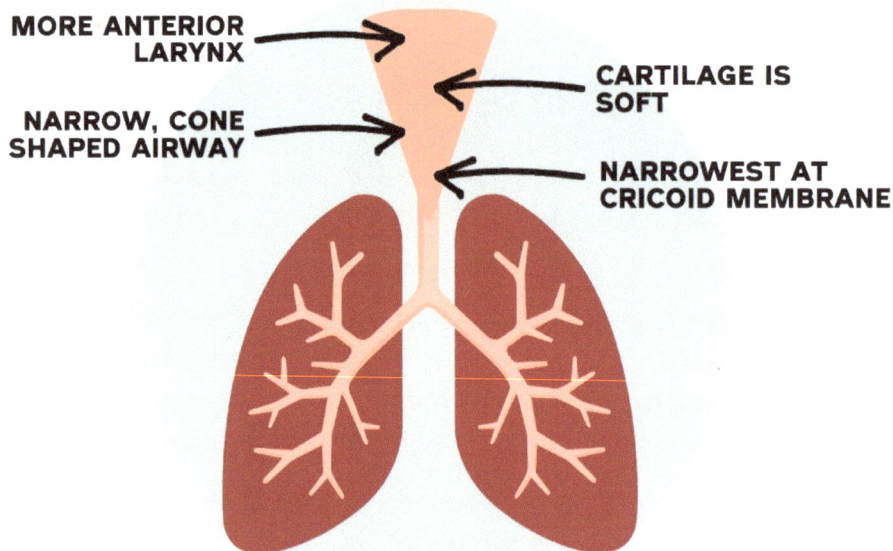

MORE ANTERIOR LARYNX

CARTILAGE IS SOFT

NARROW, CONE SHAPED AIRWAY

NARROWEST AT CRICOID MEMBRANE

Surfactant Administration[5]
- **Dose: 3mL/kg via ETT**
- **Must be given EARLY to be effective**
  - **Associated with a greater improvement and decreased need for ventilatory support**

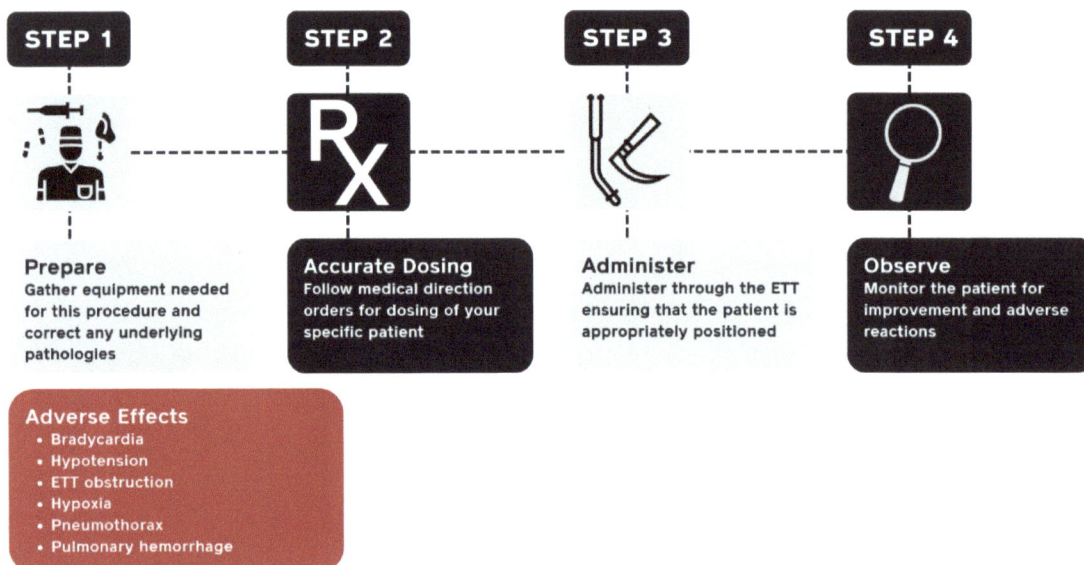

STEP 1

Prepare
Gather equipment needed for this procedure and correct any underlying pathologies

STEP 2

R̶X

Accurate Dosing
Follow medical direction orders for dosing of your specific patient

STEP 3

Administer
Administer through the ETT ensuring that the patient is appropriately positioned

STEP 4

Observe
Monitor the patient for improvement and adverse reactions

Adverse Effects
- Bradycardia
- Hypotension
- ETT obstruction
- Hypoxia
- Pneumothorax
- Pulmonary hemorrhage

Neonatal pathologies

Meconium Aspiration Syndrome
- Presents with:
  - Atelectasis
  - Persistent Pulmonary Hypertension (PPH)
    - Delays fetal to neonatal circulatory transition
  - Pneumonitis
  - Pneumothorax
  - Treatment
    - Monitor for respiratory distress, treat with PPV, high PEEP, or surfactant

Respiratory Distress Syndrome (RDS)[8]
- Surfactant deficiency related to preterm delivery
  - Decreased compliance
  - Atelectasis
  - V/Q mismatch
  - Tachypnea
  - Increased work of breathing
  - Ground-glass chest radiography
- Treatment:
  - Oxygen administration
  - CPAP (6-8cmH$_2$O)
  - Intubation and mechanical ventilation
  - IV fluids
  - IV antibiotics

Gastroschisis[8]
- Herniation of abdominal contents through abdominal wall
  - Usually on right side of umbilicus
- Pre-hospital: treat like an abdominal evisceration
  - Abdominal bag
    - Moisture, temperature, and germ barrier
  - Gastric decompression via orogastric tube
  - NPO
  - Side-lying position
  - IV antibiotics
  - Definitive care: surgical repair

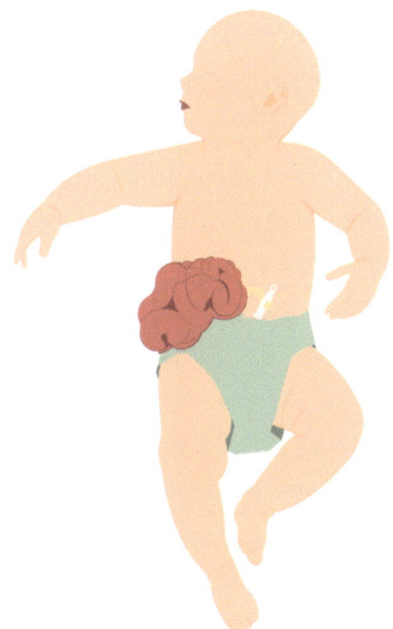

Omphalocele[8]
- Protrusion of viscera attached to the umbilical cord
- Pre-hospital: treat like an abdominal evisceration
  - Abdominal bag
    - Thermoregulation
    - Moisture
    - Germ barrier
  - NPO
  - Maintenance fluids
  - Gastric decompression via orogastric tube
- Definitive care: surgical repair
- Associated with congenital defects like diaphragmatic hernia

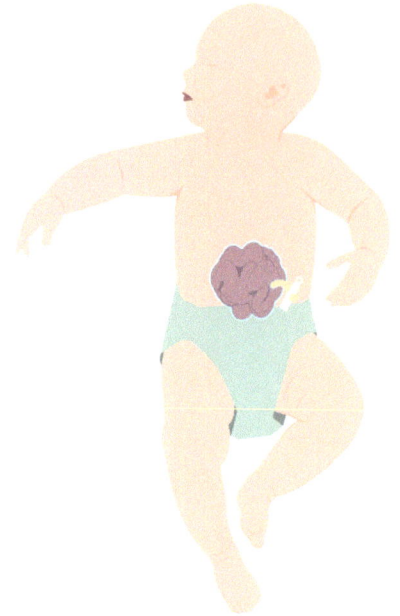

Congenital Diaphragmatic Hernia[8]
- Diaphragm fails to close during prenatal development, abdominal contents present in thorax
  - Scaphoid abdomen
  - Bowel sounds over chest
- Risk of pulmonary hypoplasia and underdevelopment of pulmonary vasculature
  - May lead to pulmonary hypertension
- Transport treatment
  o Gastric tube
  o Intubation
  o Fluid boluses
  o Inotropes
  o Antibiotics
- Definitive treatment
  o Surgical repair

Intestinal Malrotation and Volvulus[1]
- Malrotation: twisting of small bowel over on itself resulting in obstruction
- Volvulus: strangulation of bowel from malrotation
- Symptoms
  - Vomiting, diarrhea/hematochezia, or constipation
  - Drawing legs up into chest
  - Abdominal pain, abdominal distension
  - Rectal bleeding
  - Failure to thrive
  - Inconsolable crying and irritation

Intussusception
- Intestine telescopes into itself resulting in intestinal hypoperfusion and ischemia
  - Rare in neonates
- Most commonly occurs at the level of the ileo-colic junction

- Treatment: air bolus to reduce intussusception or surgery

Primary and Secondary Apnea[1]
- A pause in respirations >20 seconds
- Associated with cyanosis, pallor, hypotonia, or bradycardia

PRIMARY:
  - The initial response to asphyxia
  - Responds well to stimulation and oxygen supply

SECONDARY:
  - Occurs after a few gasping breaths
  - Responds exclusively to assisted ventilation and oxygen

Pneumothorax
- Simple vs. Tension
- Symptoms:
  - Hypoxia, cyanosis
  - Increased oxygen requirement, respiratory rate, and work of breathing
  - Agitation
  - Bradycardia/Tachycardia
  - Hypotension (severe pneumothorax)
- Diagnostic tool: transillumination or chest x-ray

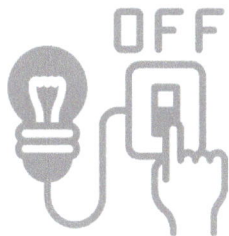

Reduce ambient light

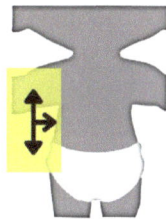

Place transilluminator at 3rd-4th ICS at posterior axillary line and angle light toward the xiphoid process

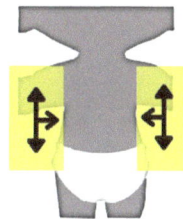

Procedure should be performed bilaterally to confirm findings

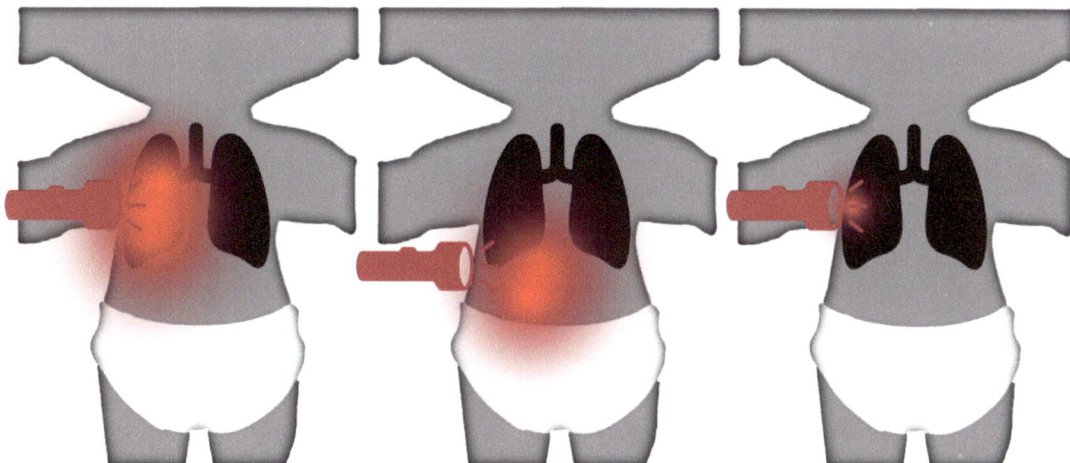

1: Pneumothorax, 2: False positive due to low placement of flashlight, 3: No pneumothorax

- **Treatment**
  - **Needle thoracostomy or chest tube**
  - **Intubation can cause and/or worsen pneumothorax**
  - **Needle thoracostomy and chest tube placement:**

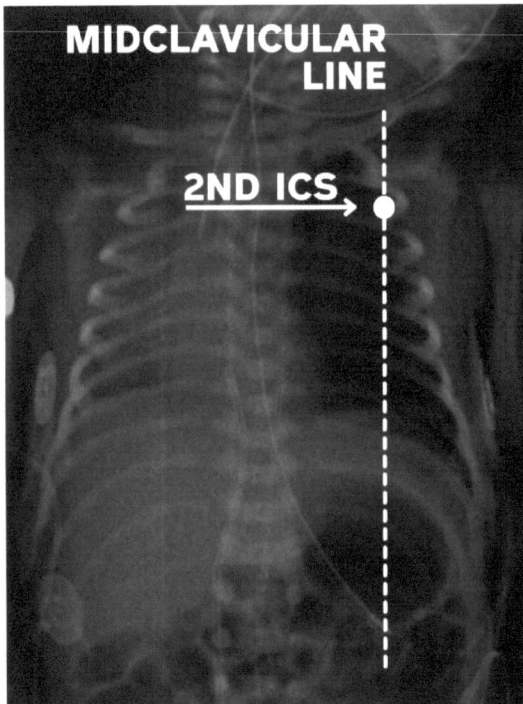

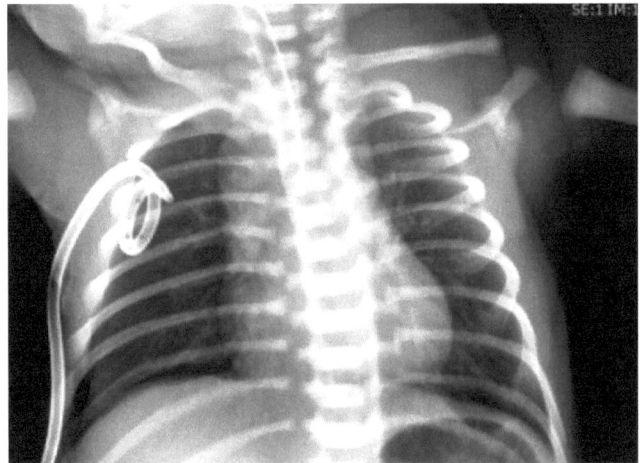

Congenital heart defects

Transposition of the Great Vessels
- Aorta and pulmonary artery are swapped

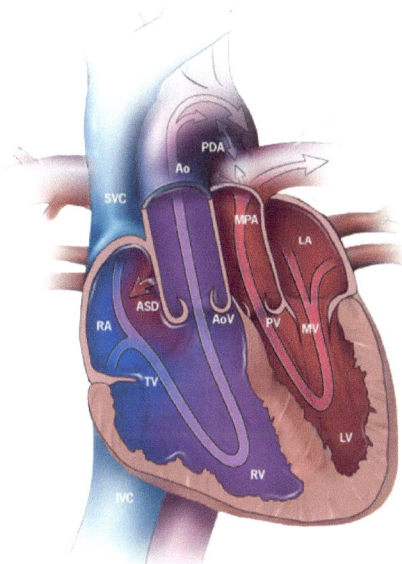

Coarctation of the Aorta
Narrowing of the aorta
- Signs/ Symptoms
  - Pale skin
  - Irritability
  - Significant diaphoresis
  - Increased work of breathing
  - Difficulty feeding

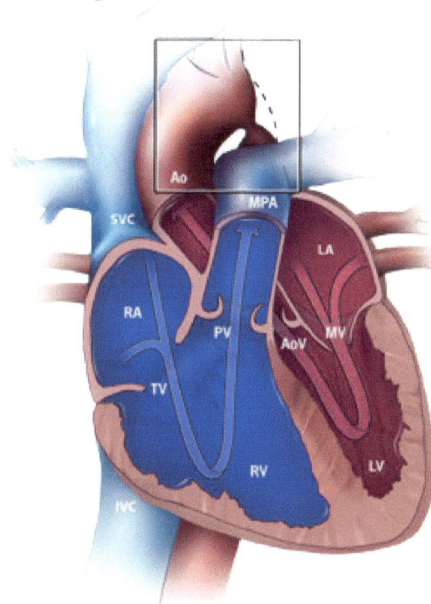

Ventricular Septal Defect (VSD)
- **Blood flows from left ventricle to right ventricle through opening in ventricular septal wall**

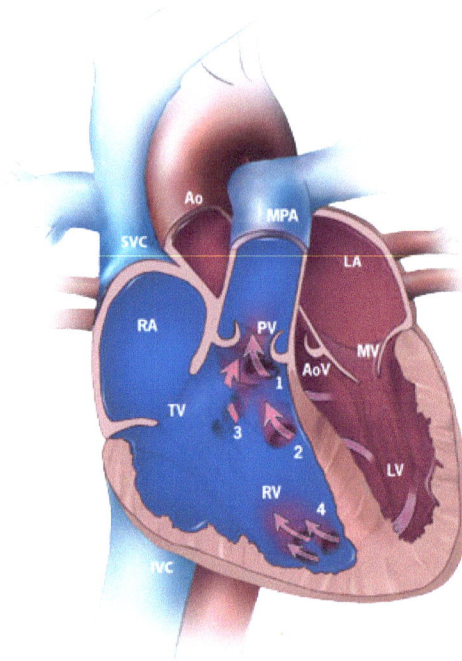

Image: CDC

Atrial Septal Defect
- **Blood flows between left and right atrium through opening in atrial septal wall**

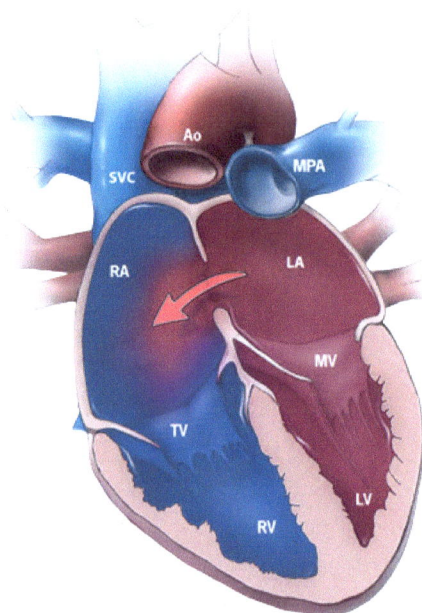

Image: CDC

Hypoplastic Left Heart Syndrome
- **Abnormally small left ventricle**

- **Aortic and mitral valve stenosis**
- **Heart failure, cyanosis, failure to thrive**

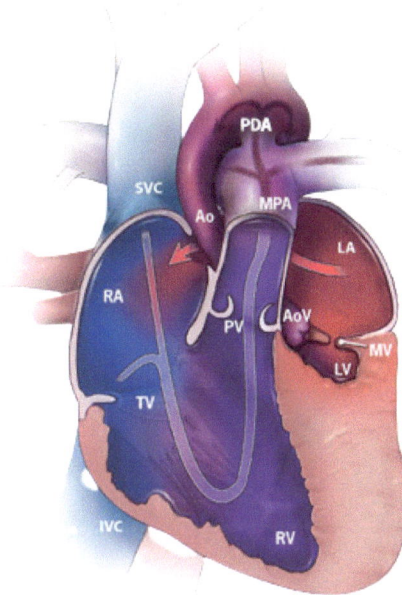

Image: CDC

Patent Ductus Arteriosus (PDA)[1]
- **Vessel that allows blood to flow from aorta to the pulmonary artery**
  - **Normal in fetal circulation, typically closes 12-24 hours after delivery**
    - **Administer indomethacin to facilitate closure**
  - **After closure, it becomes the ligamentum arteriosum**
- **Cyanotic heart defects depend on PDA**
  - **Administer prostaglandin to maintain patency**

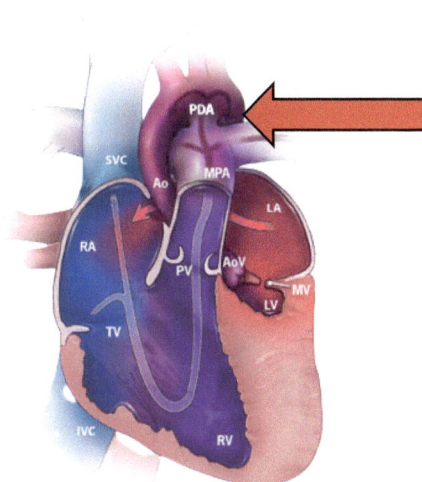

Image: CDC

Tetralogy of Fallot[11]
Concurrence of:

- **Pulmonary Stenosis**
- **Right Ventricular Hypertrophy**
- **Overriding Aorta**
- **Ventricular Septal Defect**
- **"Tet Spells" are characterized by sudden cyanosis and syncope**
- **Treat with knees to chest, morphine, or fentanyl**
- **If knees to chest/morphine does not resolve tet spell perform RSI, intubate, 100% FiO$_2$**

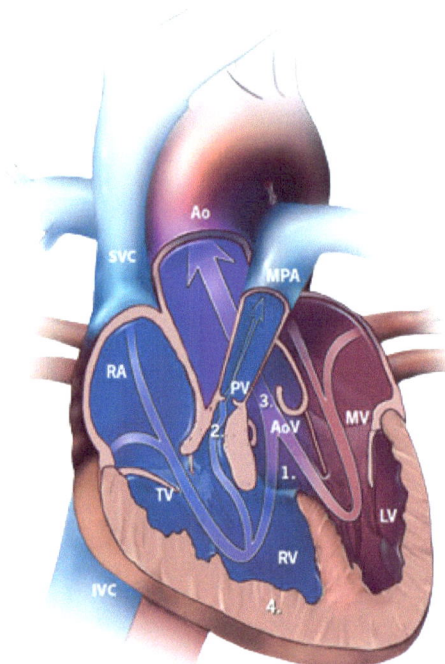

Image: CDC

Persistent Pulmonary Hypertension (PPHN)

- Persistence in elevated pressures in pulmonary vasculature after birth
- Exact cause is unknown
- Suspected causes include:
    - Meconium aspiration
    - Asphyxia
    - Pneumonia
    - Hypothermia
    - Sepsis
    - Likely will have a <u>patent foramen ovale</u> and <u>patent ductus arteriosus</u>

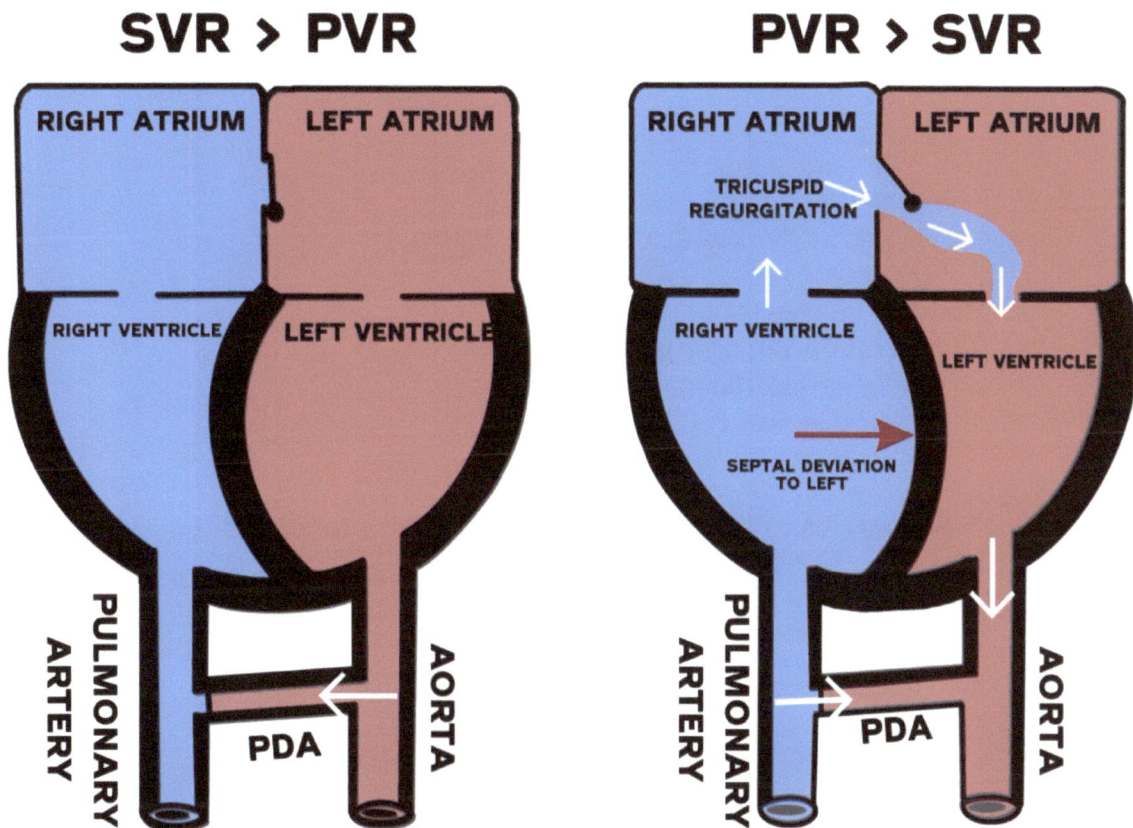

Digitalis

- Cardiac glycoside with positive inotropic and negative chronotropic actions
- Dose: 15-40mcg/kg over 24 hours

Choanal Atresia[1]
- Structural obstruction of nasopharynx requiring surgical repair to create passageway that facilitates nose breathing
- Transport considerations: place oropharyngeal airway or intubate

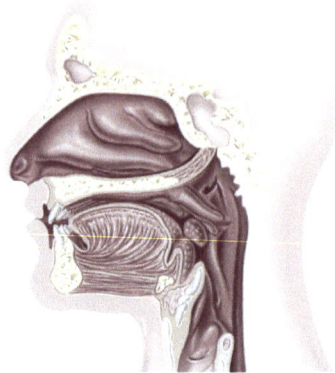

Pierre Robin Syndrome[1]
- Cluster of anomalies that cause airway obstruction
  - Small chin
  - Posterior tongue
  - Treatment during transport
    - Prone positioning
    - Oral airway

Neonatal Sepsis

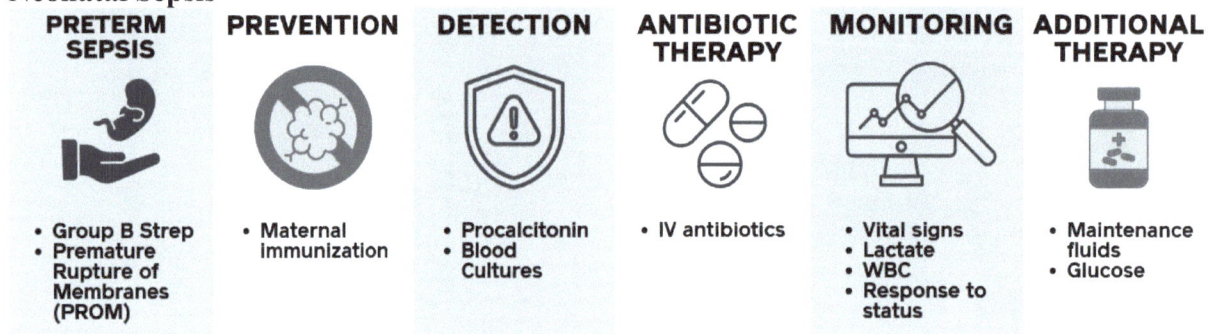

PRETERM SEPSIS	PREVENTION	DETECTION	ANTIBIOTIC THERAPY	MONITORING	ADDITIONAL THERAPY
• Group B Strep • Premature Rupture of Membranes (PROM)	• Maternal immunization	• Procalcitonin • Blood Cultures	• IV antibiotics	• Vital signs • Lactate • WBC • Response to status	• Maintenance fluids • Glucose

Seizures[8]
- Indicative of an underlying pathology
  - Hypoglycemia, hypoxia, electrolyte derangement, opioid withdrawal, intraventricular hemorrhage
- Signs:
  - Bicycling of legs
  - Lip smacking and tongue thrusting
  - Eye fluttering, rhythmic blinking, eye deviation
  - Hypoxia
- Often missed, misattributed as infant sleeping

Hypoxic Ischemic Encephalopathy

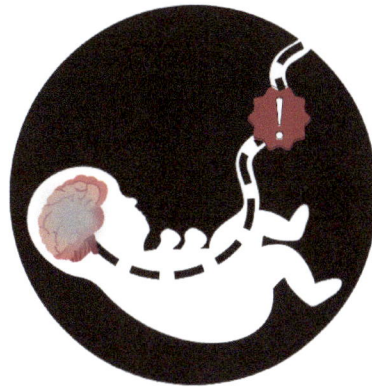

HYPOXIC= SHORTAGE OF OXYGEN

ISCHEMIC= LACK OF BLOOD FLOW

ENCEPHALOPATHY= THE RESULTANT BRAIN DAMAGE

ANY INJURY, INSULT, OR COMPLICATION THAT INTERRUPTS THE FLOW OF OXYGENATED BLOOD CAN RESULT IN HIE

Fluid Boluses
- 10mL/kg for neonatal resuscitation
- If unable to initiate IV line, consider umbilical vein catheterization
  - Normal Cord
    - 2 arteries (thick walled, inferior position)
    - 1 vein (thin walled, typically superior)

    Be mindful of post-medication flushes, risk for overload

Umbilical Vein Catheterization

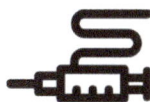

Cleanse umbilical stump and loosely tie with umbilical tape to control bleeding

Transverse cut stump 1-2 cm from skin to expose vasculature

Identify the larger, thin-walled vein and two smaller, thick-walled arteries

Securely holding stump, insert 5 French catheter or 20g IV catheter (without needle) into vein, advance 1-2cm past initial blood return

Attach stopcock to tubing, secure with occlusive dressing, and flush line

Neonatal Ventilation Pearls

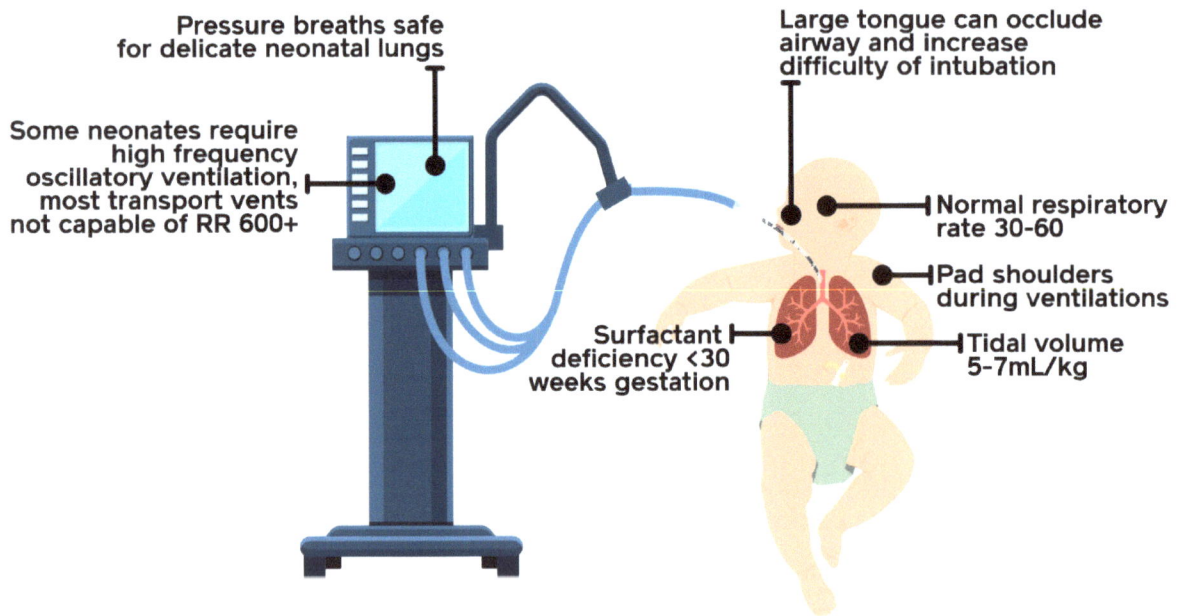

Pressure breaths safe for delicate neonatal lungs

Some neonates require high frequency oscillatory ventilation, most transport vents not capable of RR 600+

Large tongue can occlude airway and increase difficulty of intubation

Normal respiratory rate 30-60

Pad shoulders during ventilations

Surfactant deficiency <30 weeks gestation

Tidal volume 5-7mL/kg

question:

1. An appropriate fluid bolus for a neonate weighing 1957 grams is:

    a. 20mL D5NS
    b. 40mL NS
    c. 20mL NS
    d. 10mL D5NS

Chapter 16 citations:

1. Mejia, A. (2022). Critical Care Transport (3rd ed.). Jones and Bartlett Learning.
2. Changes in the newborn at birth. (n.d.). https://medlineplus.gov/ency/article/002395.htm
3. The Fetal Circulation - Shunts - Fetal haemoglobin. (2022, May 3). TeachMePhysiology. https://teachmephysiology.com/reproductive-system/fetal-physiology/fetal-circulation/
4. Surfactant replacement therapy for neonates. (2013, August). Safer care.vic.gov.au. https://www.safercare.vic.gov.au/clinical-guidance/neonatal/surfactant-replacement-therapy-for-neonates
5. Figure 1 | Pediatric Research. (2014, October 10). Nature. https://www.nature.com/articles/pr2014161/figures/1?error=cookies_not_supported&code=779ea7a5-6d1b-4f51-837a-1f03f118f1ff
6. 6. American Academy of Pediatrics (AAP), American Heart Association, Md, G. W. M., & Nnp-Bc, Z. J. R. M. (2021). Textbook of Neonatal Resuscitation (NRP) (Eighth). American Academy of Pediatrics.
7. 7. ASTNA. (2017). Patient Transport: Principles and Practice. Mosby.
8. 8. Pneumothorax and Transillumination. (2021, August 21). cahs.health.wa.gov.au. https://www.cahs.health.wa.gov.au/~/media/HSPs/CAHS/Documents/Health-Professionals/Neonatology-guidelines/Pneumothorax-and-Transillumination.pdf?thn=0
9. 9. Neonatology On Call Problems. (n.d.). http://www.neonatologybook.com/neonataloncallproblems.html
10. 10. Tetralogy of Fallot (TOF). (2022, May 5). Johns Hopkins Medicine. https://www.hopkinsmedicine.org/health/conditions-and-diseases/tetralogy-of-fallot-tof

Chapter 17: Pediatric critical care

Foundations of Pediatric Critical Care

Pediatric Assessment Triangle[12]

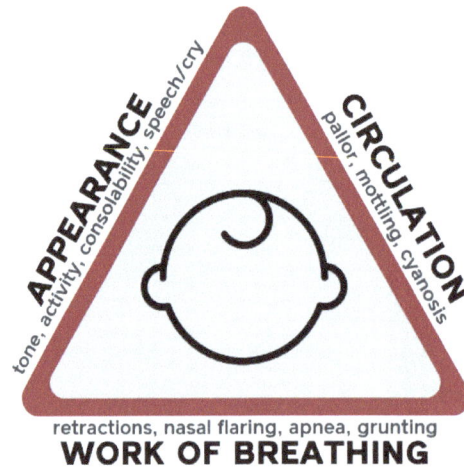

retractions, nasal flaring, apnea, grunting
WORK OF BREATHING

Work of Breathing[9]
- Increased work of breathing takes up 40% of a child's cardiac output
- Increased work of breathing leads to dehydration

Normal Pediatric Vital Signs[12]

	Weight in lbs	Weight in kgs	Resp Rate	Heart Rate	Systolic BP
Preterm (<37 wks)	1.5-5.5	0.7-2.5	50-70	120-180	40-60
Newborn (37-42 wks)	5.5-9	2.5-4	40-60	100-170	50-70
Neonate (1-28 days)	7.5-11	3.4-5	30-50	90-160	60-80
Infant (1-12 months)	10-22	4.5-10	25-40	80-160	70-100
Toddler (1-3 years)	22-32	10-14.5	20-30	80-130	70-110
Preschooler (3-5 years)	32-42	14.5-19	20-30	80-110	80-110
School Age (6-12 years)	42-90	19-41	20-24	75-100	80-120
Adolescent (>13 years)	>90	>41	12-20	60-90	94-130

IV Fluid Boluses[15]
- Generally: 100 mL of fluid is needed per 100 calories the kid uses
- Bolus dose: 20 mL/kg (up to three times)
  - Normal saline

Pediatric Maintenance Fluid
- **Should be glucose containing solution (D5NS, D5 1/2NS)**

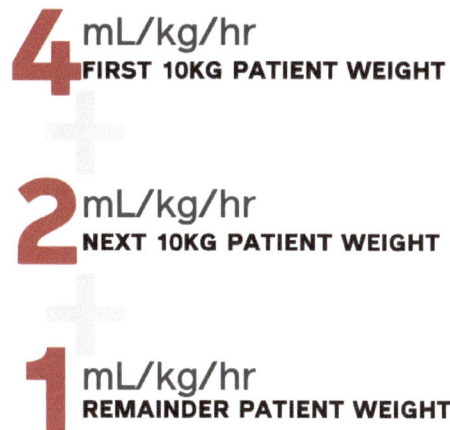

4 mL/kg/hr
FIRST 10KG PATIENT WEIGHT

2 mL/kg/hr
NEXT 10KG PATIENT WEIGHT

1 mL/kg/hr
REMAINDER PATIENT WEIGHT

General Pediatric Pharmacology[9]
- **Pediatrics have large amounts of adipose tissue**
  - **Fat is poorly perfused so use caution in IM meds**
- **May require higher loading doses because of plasma concentrations**
- **IO rate of absorption is comparable to IV**
- **Consider nebulized and intranasal pain medication control**

Pediatric Airway & Pulmonary Management

Oxygen[9]
- **Pulse oximetry is required**
- **ABG is of limited value**
- **Kids tolerate hypercarbia extremely well**
- **THE BASICS WILL NOT FAIL YOU**

Airflow[9]
- **Children have narrower airways**
- **Narrower airways may require higher pressures to diffuse oxygen**
  - **Heliox**
- **Pressure diffusion gradient is proportional to the gas flow rate**

Upper Airway Obstruction[9]
- **Hallmark sign is inspiratory stridor**
- **Serious obstruction may occur without stridor**
- **Upper airway is narrow in smaller children**
- **Narrowest part of airway is the cricoid ring**

Congenital Upper Airway Pathologies[2,9]
- Craniofacial dysmorphism with midface hypoplasia
  - Pierre Robin Syndrome
  - Treacher Collins Syndrome
  - Choanal atresia

Laryngomalacia[9]
- Most common cause of stridor in infancy
- Floppy larynx
- Usually normalizes over time

Laryngotracheobronchitis (Croup)[9]
- Barking cough and loud inspiratory stridor
- "Steeple sign" on x-ray
- Usually has preceding respiratory infection
- Treated with racemic epinephrine
  - L-epinephrine or epinephrine alternatives
  - May cause tachycardia
    - VERY well-tolerated, do NOT withhold

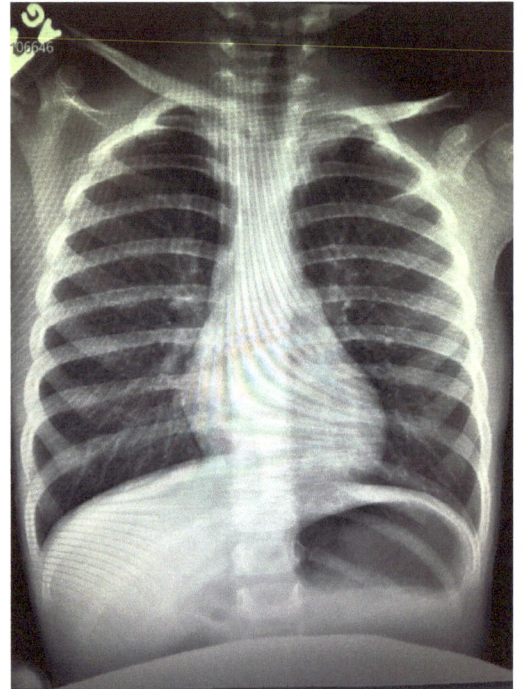

Bacterial Tracheitis[9]
- Most common cause of acute infectious upper airway respiratory failure
- Purulent secretions noted on intubation
- Bacterial superinfection in patients with viral croup

Epiglottitis[9]
- Acute, life-threatening airway compromise
- Usually Flu B
- "Thumbprint" sign on x-ray
- Occurs at any age
- Classic presentation:
  - Stridor
  - Fever
  - Rapidly progressing dyspnea

Lower Airway: Asthma[4,9]

- Often poorly controlled in children
- Have a low threshold for more intensive treatment
- Avoid intubation if possible
  - Indications for intubation in peds asthma:
    - Fatigue
    - Altered mental status
- Mechanical ventilation: Extend e-time

Bronchiolitis[9]

- Most common cause is RSV
- Airway obstruction
- Decreased compliance
- Ciliary dysfunction and airway debris
- Initial upper respiratory symptoms
  - 48-72 hours later: lower airway symptoms
- Treated with humidified oxygen and hydration

High-Flow Nasal Cannula[6]

- Dead space
  - Airway space not taking part in gas exchange
- Oxygen dilution
  - Rebreathed carbon dioxide
  - Oropharyngeal air has around 11% O_2
- Heated and humidified O_2
  - Improves mucus clearance
  - Decreases airway inflammation
  - Better compliance
  - Reduced caloric expenditure

Non-Invasive Ventilation[11]

- Indications: respiratory failure
  - Dyspnea and supplemental oxygen required to keep SpO_2 >92%
  - $PaCO_2$ >50 with arterial pH <7.35*
- Three physiologic benefits
  - Decreases work of breathing
  - Maintains airway patency
  - Alveolar recruitment

The Pediatric Airway[9]
- Floppy and U-shaped epiglottis
- Glottis more anterior and higher
- Narrow cricoid ring
- More flexible trachea
- Tongue is giant relative to other structures
- Oral space is limited

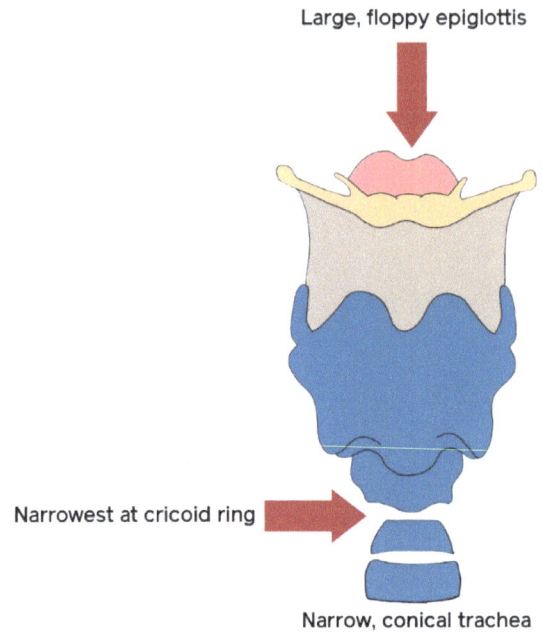

Large, floppy epiglottis

Narrowest at cricoid ring

Narrow, conical trachea

Pediatric Intubation[9]
- Indication is hypoxia
  - Hypercarbia is only an indication for intubation if there is hypoxemia
- Desaturations are very common and sudden
- Hypotension common with RSI drugs
- IV fluids should be administered prior to intubation

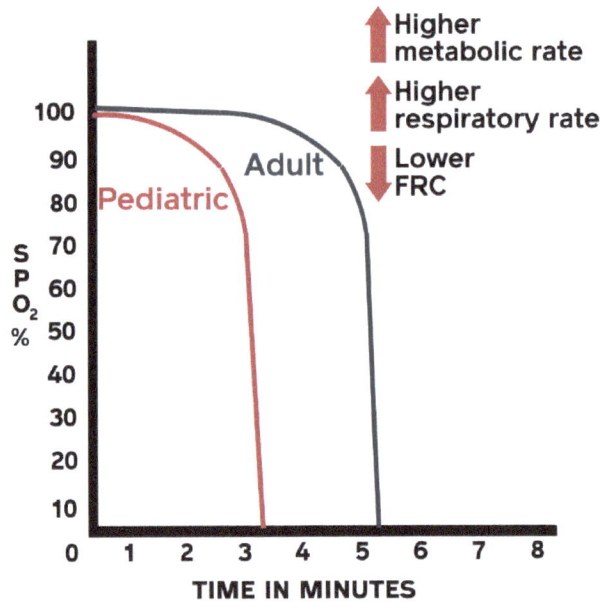

Higher metabolic rate

Higher respiratory rate

Lower FRC

Adult

Pediatric

SPO$_2$ %

TIME IN MINUTES

Invasive Ventilation[9,10]
- Children more susceptible to dead space
  - Adjust for dead space: tidal volume
- Risk of barotrauma
  - Lung protection strategy
- Reduce FiO$_2$ as quickly as feasible
- Positive pressure → hypotension

Febrile Seizures

- The rate of temperature increase is the provocative factor in febrile seizures
- 1° change >37° increases heart rate by 10
- Does not require further workup
  - Increased likelihood of additional febrile seizures up to age 5

Pediatric Trauma

Hypovolemic Shock[3,8]
- Traumatic shock in the pediatric patient is most commonly due to hypovolemia
- First sign of compensation is tachycardia
- Kids remain in compensated shock for quite some time
- Minor blood loss in an adult can have major consequences for a child

Shock Resuscitation[3,8,9]
- Higher fluid resuscitation requirements
  - Bolus dose is 20 mL/kg
  - Kids need fluid at 3x the blood loss
- Isotonic crystalloid is resuscitative solution of choice
  - Blood reserved if no response to crystalloid
- TXA is safe and effective
- Vasopressors are not appropriate for shock resuscitation due to hypovolemia

Pediatric Neurotrauma[3]
- Head injuries and skull fractures quite common
- Most spinal injuries occur in cervical region
- SCIWORA more commonly seen in children
- Epidural hematoma presents differently
  - More common due to edges of skull fracture causing lacerations
  - May present anywhere in the skull
  - Typically venous vs. arterial

Waddell's Triad: Pedestrian Accidents[13]

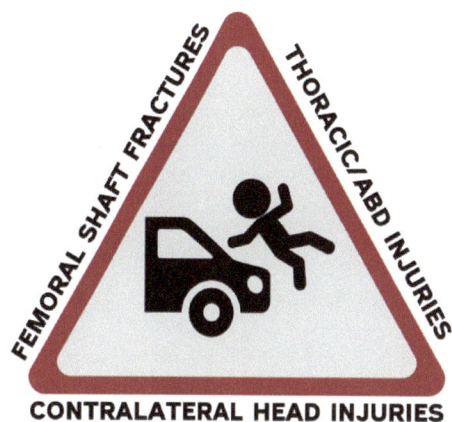

FEMORAL SHAFT FRACTURES
THORACIC/ABD INJURIES
CONTRALATERAL HEAD INJURIES

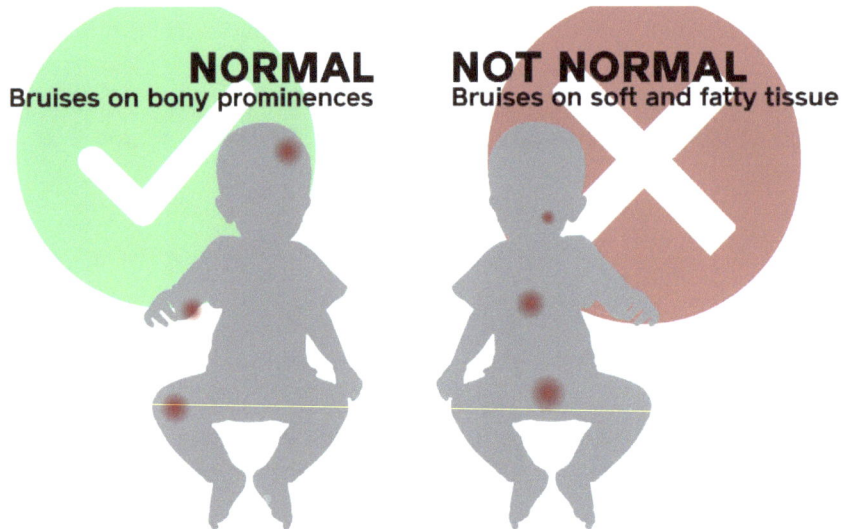

NORMAL
Bruises on bony prominences

NOT NORMAL
Bruises on soft and fatty tissue

Non-Accidental Trauma[1,14]
- **Pattern of injuries**
- **Sexually transmitted infections never normal**
- **"Shaken Baby Syndrome"**
  - **Intracerebral hemorrhages of all types**
  - **Multiple sites of hemorrhage**
    - **Retinal hemorrhage classic Shaken Baby Syndrome**
  - **Diffuse axonal injury**
  - **Skull fractures**

Special Needs & High-tech Kids

Special Needs Considerations[2]
- **If you are being called, something is wrong**
- **Utilize the parents, they are experts**
- **Consider contacting their specialist or medical command at their specialty hospital**
- **Admission rate is around 50%**
  - **Most common: respiratory**
  - **Gastrointestinal**
  - **Neuro**

Ventriculoperitoneal (VP) Shunt
- **Treatment for increased CSF in congenital hydrocephalus**
    - **VP shunts frequently malfunction**
- **Cerebral spinal fluid buildup increases ICP**
    - **High-pitched cry**
    - **Vomiting, abdominal distention**
    - **Sun-setting eyes**
    - **Bulging fontanels**
    - **Seizures**

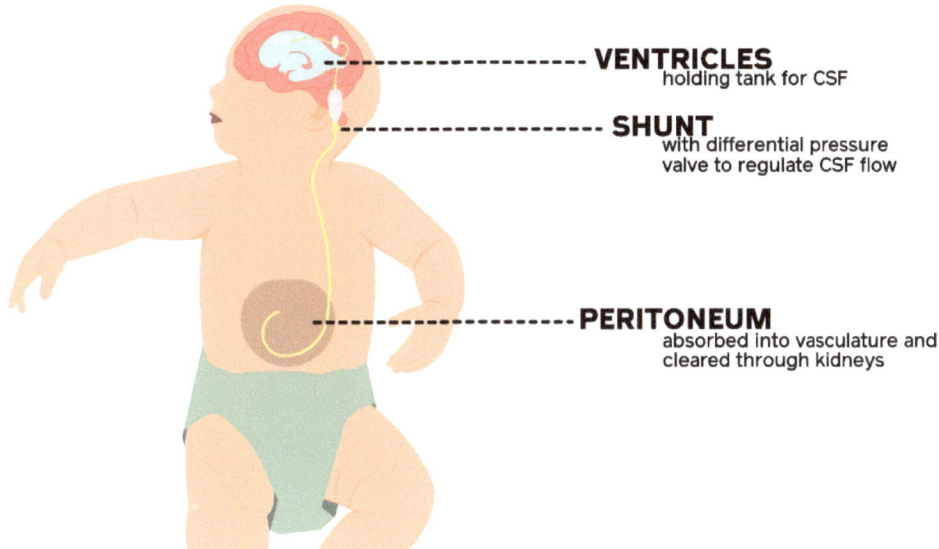

VENTRICLES
holding tank for CSF

SHUNT
with differential pressure
valve to regulate CSF flow

PERITONEUM
absorbed into vasculature and
cleared through kidneys

Questions:

The first sign of compensation in the pediatric patient with hemorrhagic shock is:

    a. **Reduction of SBP by 15%**
    b. **Increased respiratory rate**
    c. **Sustained tachycardia**
    d. **Narrowing pulse pressure**

Which of the following findings in the pediatric patient with respiratory distress is the most IMMEDIATELY alarming?

    a. **PO_2 70 mmHg**
    b. **SpO_2 84%**
    c. **PCO_2 80 mmHg**
    d. **SvO_2 84%**

Chapter 17 Citations:

1. Cianci P, D'Apolito V, Moretti A, Barbagallo M, Paci S, Carbone MT, Lubrano R, Urbino A, Dionisi Vici C, Memo L, Zampino G, La Marca G, Villani A, Corsello G, Selicorni A; Italian Society of Pediatrics (SIP); Italian Society of Pediatric Genetic Diseases and Congenital Disabilities (SIMGePed) the Italian Society of Pediatric Emergency Medicine (SIMEUP); Italian Society For The Study Of Inborn Metabolic Disorders And Newborn Screening (SIMMENS) and Members of Italian Network. Children with special health care needs attending emergency department in Italy: analysis of 3479 cases. Ital J Pediatr. 2020 Nov 23;46(1):173. doi: 10.1186/s13052-020-00937-x. PMID: 33228805; PMCID: PMC7685641.

2. Elias, E., Murphy, N. (2012). Home Care of Children and Youth with Complex Health Care Needs and Technology Dependencies. Pediatrics. doi:10.1542/peds.2012-0606

3. Figaji AA. Anatomical and Physiological Differences between Children and Adults Relevant to Traumatic Brain Injury and the Implications for Clinical Assessment and Care. Front Neurol. 2017 Dec 14;8:685. doi: 10.3389/fneur.2017.00685. PMID: 29312119; PMCID: PMC5735372.

4. Fox, Sean. (2015). Mechanical Ventilation for Severe Asthma. Available: https://pedemmorsels.com/mechanical-ventilation-severe-asthma/

Chapter 18: Study tips

Study Strategies

Break your study sessions into 25-minute blocks.
Take advantage of your breaks! Use them to reset your brain.

1

PREPARE.
Gather your materials. Find a study zone. Silence or DND, ignore all distractions.

2

STUDY.
Set your timer for 25 minutes. Focus all your energy on studying only for those minutes.

3

BREAK TIME.
Set your timer for a 5 minute break. Get up. Stretch. Water. Snack. Fuel your brain.

4

STUDY TIME.
Back to the grind. Set another 25 minute timer and repeat steps two and three.

5

REPEAT.
Continue the 25 minute – 5 minute break pattern for a total of four (4) rounds.

6

LONGER BREAK.
After 4th round take a 30 minute timed break and enjoy! Repeat if studying more.

If you are stuck on a topic, please reach out to us via our website at www.ImpactEMS.com or on social media platforms where our instructors interact with our learners on a regular basis!

Answer key

Chapter 1: 1. B, 2. C, 3. C, 4. D

Chapter 2: 1. Uncompensated Respiratory Acidosis, 2. Uncompensated Metabolic Acidosis, 3. Fully Compensated Respiratory Acidosis, 4. Partially Compensated Respiratory Acidosis, 5. Uncompensated Metabolic Alkalosis, 6. Uncompensated Respiratory Acidosis, 7. Compensated Respiratory Acidosis

Chapter 3: 1. This patient likely has a pulmonary embolism secondary to venous stasis after surgery. Transport priorities include administration of high flow oxygen and hemodynamic support. This patient requires rapid transport to a facility capable of administering thrombolytics or performing clot retrieval. 2. B, 3. D

Chapter 4: 1. A, 2. B, 3. B, 4. B, Bonus: Tension pneumothorax

Chapter 5: Your differential for this patient should include liver failure. This patient requires blood administration, and the transport providers should be exceptionally careful to prevent bleeding with this patient due to low clotting factors. After administration of five units of packed red blood cells, the patient's hemoglobin should be in the ballpark of seven with an expected hematocrit of 21%. The clinician should also expect severe electrolyte derangements and should assess lab values and replace electrolytes appropriately.

Chapter 6: 1. D, 3. C

Chapter 7: 1. D, 2. D

Chapter 8: 1. C, 2. C

Chapter 9: 1. A, 2. A

Chapter 10: 1. B, 2. B

Chapter 11: 1. D

Chapter 12: 1. This patient likely has a subarachnoid hemorrhage, which would appear on a CT scan with a starfish pattern. The blood pressure should be treated with an esmolol or nicardipine drip to target a systolic blood pressure less than 160. 2. A

Chapter 13: 1. B, 2. A, 3. A, 4. D

Chapter 14: 1. C

Chapter 15: 1. A, 2. D, 3. This strip reveals variable decelerations, which is concerning for cord compression. In the transport setting, the provider should check the vagina for a prolapsed cord, and if there is no prolapsed cord, administer a fluid bolus, turn the mother on her left side, and placed the mother on high flow oxygen via nonrebreather.

Chapter 16: 1. C

Chapter 17: 1. C, 2. B